Rocks in My Pockets

Rocks in My Pockets

Travels with Dad

Claudia Crosetti

iUniverse, Inc.

New York   Lincoln   Shanghai

Rocks in My Pockets
Travels with Dad

Copyright © 2007 by Claudia L. Crosetti

iUniverse books may be ordered through booksellers or by contacting:

iUniverse
2021 Pine Lake Road, Suite 100
Lincoln, NE 68512
www.iuniverse.com
1-800-Authors (1-800-288-4677)

The views expressed in this work are solely those of the author and do not necessarily reflect the views of the publisher, and the publisher hereby disclaims any responsibility for them.

ISBN: 978-0-595-43844-0

Printed in the United States of America

This book is dedicated to my family and to the memory of my teammates whose strength of spirit remains close to my heart: Laura Evans, Andrea Martin, Claudia Berryman-Shaefer and Roger Evans.

Foreword

When I returned from Italy it took three days before I could face the streets of my hometown. What was it about the Italian culture that so captivated my soul and spirit? Determined to keep the experience alive, I began to chronicle my impressions of our daily wanderings. Each day as I wrote, I thought of one of my sisters—the one who had yet to visit a European country. How exactly would I describe to her the pulsating beat of the vital downtowns, the maze-like configurations of cobbled streets, the exquisite architecture and the simple, yet delicious, food? And so the layers of my story unfolded—my travels with Dad. The muses, however, were not fully satisfied with my romp through the country of my ancestors: they led me down a second path—one of reflection. Plunging me back in time, images of my childhood and several life-changing events came streaming into my consciousness, unleashing yet another journey altogether—and one that now lies within.

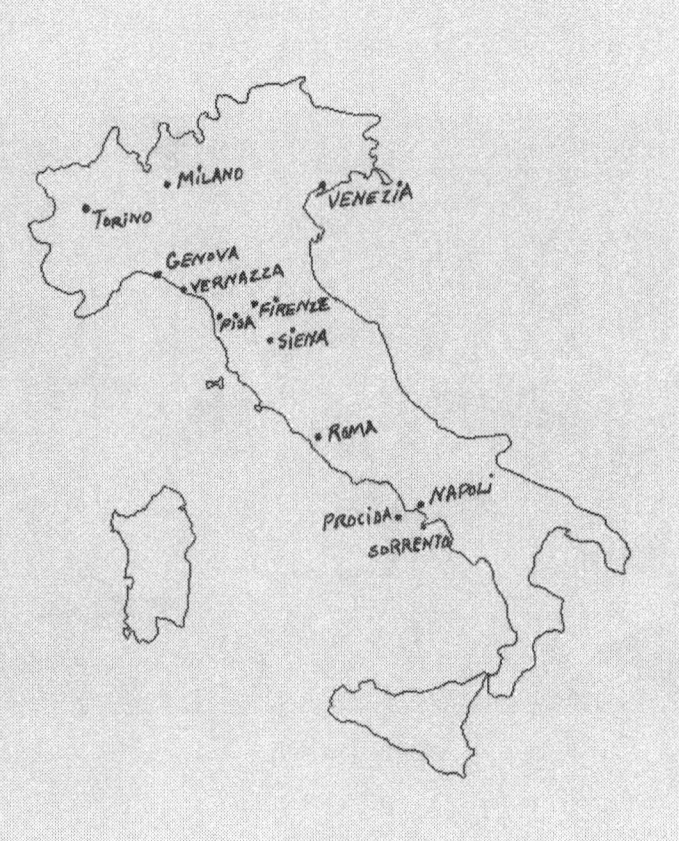

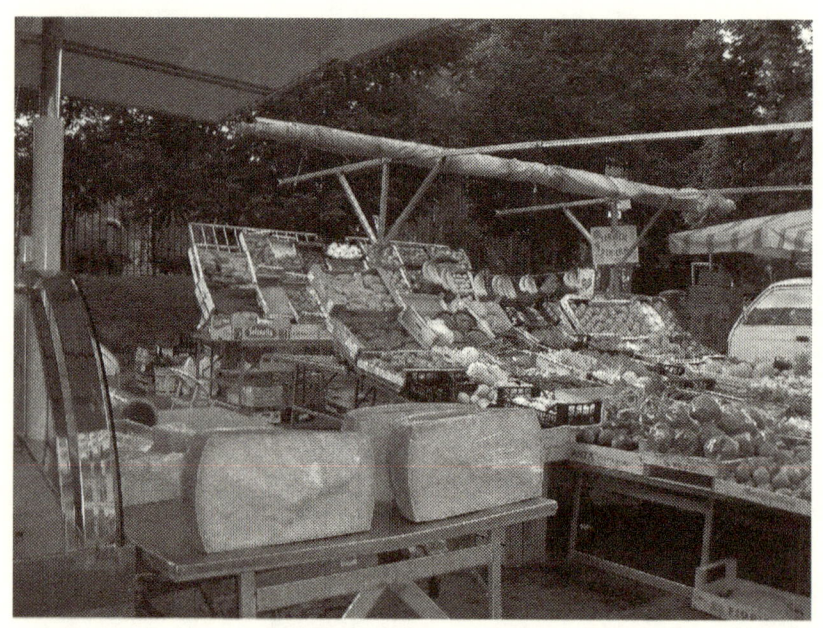

Milano—Produce Stand

Milano

26 Settembre

"Let's not take the taxi to our hotel, Dad! Let's walk." From the open piazza in which we stand, cobbled streets lined with tall browned stone buildings fan out in all directions. Curving rooflines and ornate balconies accent the architecture, while statues peak from within the niches of upper stories. Twisting around, I spot a castle towering immediately behind a more modern structure. I had no idea the visual feast would begin the moment we set foot outside the train station. People are moving about us everywhere and there is no vehicle traffic whatsoever. Perhaps automobiles are blocked off from the downtown area on Sunday evenings. With packs securely tucked against our backs, we merge with the stream of promenading locals: it occurs to me we have arrived right in the midst of the Italian *passeggiatta*—the formal traditional evening stroll. Gaping up at the old, stone buildings, I practically trip over myself as I begin to notice tall, beautiful Italian men ambling slowly, seductively within the crowds. In vain, I attempt to straighten my rumpled travel shirt and run my fingers through the graying crown of my hair. While I drool at the architecture and remain overwhelmed by the masses of people in the street, Dad stays focused and stops to study the map of downtown Milano. "We shouldn't linger," he insists: "It's important we find our hotel before dark." Reorienting ourselves, we pick up the pace and head in the direction of Milano's grand gothic cathedral—the area in which Hotel Speronari is located.

Keeping stride with the promenading locals, I notice the younger generation is mostly clad in designer blue jeans; the few elders we pass are dressed neatly in more formal, conservative attire. Street vendors sell food from portable stalls and a group of musicians set up to perform at a popular intersection. We pause briefly to watch a man and his highly animated son wailing away on accordions: the boy plays eagerly like a wind-up toy, a permanent grin plastered across his face as he works hard for his tips. I wonder if every night in Milano is this lively and upbeat or is it just Sundays. We turn onto a grand cobbled thoroughfare that boasts several blocks of an outdoor photography exhibit. Spectacular aerial shots taken from far reaches of the world are displayed in huge frames. Above a sea of moving heads, I steal glimpses of the exhibit, while Dad continues ahead of me setting a mean pace. I try to not lose sight of his green wool beret that bobs up and down ahead of me in the crowd.

Drawing closer to the center of the historic downtown, we pass shops, coffee bars and a number of windows displaying women's severely pointy-toed shoes—the latest in fashion. Just as Dad is about to get out the map again, unexpectedly we turn into a spacious, cobbled square—the Piazza Del Duomo. Frozen in our tracks, the sight of Milano's gothic cathedral is a sight to behold. Her ominous exterior is flanked with marble statues residing at every level and angle. Cherubs, gods, griffins and gargoyles protect and adorn elaborate columns and niches. Across the entire depth of its rooftop, hundreds of gothic spires skewer upward, and above all else reins an angelic, Madonna of solid gold. "It's over-the-top!" I shout to Dad above the noise of the crowds gathered at the square. "It really is," he laughs "*Molto* garish …" "… and all in the name of religion." I decide early on that touring this country with my card-carrying atheist father will probably be amusing. From the corner of my eye, I can see that dad is brimming with pleasure, having just walked me through my first European city. He tells me later that at that moment, in his mind, our trip had already been a success.

With twilight upon us, we find Hotel Speronari, a three-story *albergo*, located on a quaint, cobbled street of shops and old historic buildings. At the front counter of the lobby, a robust, middle-aged Italian woman greets us in her native tongue: "Buona *Sera!* "she exudes; then switches to broken English once she discovering we speak little Italian. She hands an old-fashioned brass door key to Dad and gestures us beyond the lobby to an extremely narrow stairwell. We ascend to the second floor, where we follow a darkened hallway until we find our room. I open the door to well-lighted, narrow quarters with high ceilings and linoleum flooring. At the opposite end is a tall, shuttered window framed by translucent white flowing curtains. I choose the twin bed located near the window and dump my pack with relief upon the cool floor. Fresh air and a cacophony of city sounds ease into the room, when I throw open the shuttered windows. Two stories below me, well-dressed people duck in and out of the surrounding shops. I hang my head out in amazement of our stone surroundings. Dad and I are both beat after 20 hours of planes, trains and automobiles. My back is hot and stiff from carrying the 12 pound pack for the past hour or so. Too exhausted to explore the city tonight, we each take a hot shower and hunker down for the evening.

I remain awake for what seems like hours this evening as I try to absorb my initiation to a European city. My senses are overwhelmed from culture shock. Twenty hours ago I was among asphalt freeways and urban American sprawl. Now I lie within

*this odd environment of old stone and cobbled alleyways, sur-
rounded by a foreign tongue and feeling surprisingly alien. My
decision to visit Italy occurred last summer, following a Sunday
bike ride, over coffee with Dad and a group of friends. With no
premeditated thought, I blurted out "How would you like to go
to Italy, Dad?" At the age of 78 he was extremely fit, full of
energy, and-unlike me-seasoned at traveling in Europe. In the
late 1970's Dad spent the final two years prior to his retirement
working in the Middle East for Gulf Air. My parents took advantage of travel perks offered to any of Gulf Air's destinations,
traveling to the British Isles, Amsterdam, France and India.
Italy, however, was not one of Gulf Air's stops, so when I pitched
the idea of this trip to Dad, I had a feeling a new country—especially Italy—would appeal to him. I also knew that Mom joining
us would be out of the question, since in recent years she has
been suffering with an arthritic hip.*

*My life was feeling stagnant at the time I posed my question
to Dad. Two years earlier I had parted ways with a live-in companion. For awhile, I busied myself attending a Bachelor of Arts
weekend program in San Francisco while continuing to work at
my long-held, office administrative job at the local college.
Around that time, my home became filled with a deafening
silence that followed the death of my beloved, 20 year old cat,
Vladimir. I live in a sleepy, rural town where if you don't go
away to seek adventure and stimulation, it certainly isn't going
to come to you. By the time the words "Dad, do you want to go
to Italy?" came spewing from my lips, as if prompted from some
outer force, I realized my 50th birthday had come and gone and
I had yet to visit Europe. Enough had happened by this time in
my life to know not to put this dream off any longer. I remember
Dad had once advised me: "When you go to Europe, just pick a*

city, any city and you'll get a European experience." I think I chose Italy because of the art, the architecture, the food and no doubt because I am of half Italian descent. By the time we finished our coffee that morning, Dad was nodding his head in excitement, "Yes! I think Italy is a great idea." So out came the guide books and city maps of Italy, and the Internet searches began, as we planned our three week journey by rail and on foot through the country of my ancestors.

27 Settembre

I awake at 2:30 AM to the smell of baking brioche wafting through our open window. The smell transports me back to my childhood in Seattle. An alleyway, where we played, ran behind our three-story, middle class Victorian home. Once a week, from the kitchen of our house, the aroma of fresh baked bread drifted down the alleyway, enticing my sisters and me back inside. To this day I can smell the yeast and see the final touches of melted butter glazing over the tops of the hot, perfectly golden crusts. This morning, I drift in and out of sleep comforted by these nostalgic thoughts and the smells from the streets below. The engine of what might be a delivery truck is running and I can hear two men's voices. I am aware of my stone surroundings from last night's walk—the jumble of meandering, cobbled streets and rock-solid old buildings of downtown Milano. I contemplate the fact that Dad and I will be attached at the hip for three weeks solid. I wonder how we'll get along. He's self-sufficient, predictable and reliable—good traits, I think in a traveling companion. Still, I wonder what kind of trouble we might encounter in the coming weeks together: we barely know the language and Dad is much older than he was the last time he train-hopped through countries in Europe. I've been expecting to rely on him for guidance, now I'm somewhat daunted by my own responsi-

bilities. Our schedule is an ambitious one: Venice, Turin, Curogne, The Cinque Terre, Florence, Naples and Rome. And all without a guide. But for now, we have a full day in Milano ahead of us and I can hardly wait.

Still unadjusted to the time change, at 6:00 AM we are both fully dressed and ready to explore the *centro antico*—the old downtown. We surprise the concierge when we require the lobby door of our hotel be opened for us at this early hour. In the pitch black, we emerge into cobbled streets and dark alleyways with barely a soul in sight. Not long into our wanderings, we notice a few inviting, well-lighted coffee bars preparing to open. Large, clean windows display tables of fresh pastries—flakey *cornetto* (croissants) and fruit-filled brioche. We choose a café with an elegant mahogany and marble bar, intimate tables with white tablecloths and warm ambient lighting. A *barista* dressed in a crisp, white shirt and bow tie stands with perfect posture behind the counter, preparing for customers as he quickly shines the already-clean surface. The espresso machines are huge, sporting eight spouts. Beside them sit big cone-shaped grinders full of fresh beans and I notice there are no paper "to-go" cups in sight. Awkwardly, I manage to place our order, trying out my first Italian words: *"Due cappucini, por favore."* I gesture that we would also like two brioche. Our cappuccino is served in small, white ceramic cups with saucers and delicate silver spoons. The warm shots of espresso are served with just the right amount of steamed milk. I can't help but feel like a big American bull in a china closet as I gingerly carry our warm cups over to a table, while Dad handles the money exchange. Later, while we enjoy our quick breakfast, Dad tells me how impressed he is by the professional appearance and efficiency of service we receive from the no-nonsense *barista*. Shortly thereafter, a few early-bird working people enter and stand at the bar, while the *barista* prepares shots of espresso served in delicate white demitasse cups. The locals drink their shots rather quickly—as if they are taking medicine—then chat a bit, and move on.

We emerge from the warmth of the bar and make our way across the vacant Piazza del Duomo, passing the gothic cathedral. Her stately figures and gargoyles appear ominous—almost menacing—as they stare out at us in the dark of early morning. I can only imagine what a beautiful sight this must be at the break of dawn, the sensuous curves and various hues of marble reflected in early morning's light. As we continue away from the Duomo, we take a step up into a magnificent glass-covered galleria ... the Galleria Vittorio Emmanuelle, a 19th century version of a shopping mall. Canopied high above by leaded-glass, greenhouse-like archways, four city blocks converge into a central rotunda. We tread upon beautiful, mosaic-tiled pavement, while admiring frescos that adorn the arches and corners of the walls and ceilings. My spirits are uplifted as I stand within this solarium of sorts and savor the quiet and emptiness, knowing the galleria will be filled with people and noise in only a matter of hours. The street level of the galleria is housed with restaurants, bookstores, shops of the latest in fashion and computers and cell phones that make for an odd contrast next to the old, elegant architecture. We exit from the far side and find ourselves on the wide promenade displaying the stunning photography exhibit we walked through last night. With no one in sight we are able to leisurely examine each print in silence.

Day breaks by the time we reach Castello Sforzesco—the castle I spotted not far from the train station last night. Within the quiet of the brick walled courtyard, an elderly white-haired gentleman dressed in a rumpled gray suit, shirt and neck tie, opens a bag of dry cat food and carefully spreads its contents on a cement bench. A handful of felines dart over to him and fight off pesky pigeons as they gobble down their generous day's feeding. In another cloister of the castle grounds, a middle-aged woman who appears to work in one of the castle's offices, sets down her purse before beginning her day to feed a small colony of cats who have been patiently awaiting her arrival. It is only these cat guardians and Dad and I who seem to occupy the castle grounds this early morning. The grand, old fortification, tucked away from the bustling *centro antico* provides a safe and quiet sanctuary for *i gatti*.

In the streets of the surrounding neighborhoods vendors set up produce stands for the day. Their signs read: *Frutte e verdure*. Wooden tables display yellow bell peppers, slender purple eggplant, ripe red tomatoes, rows of citrus, and big boxes of freshly harvested mushrooms—porcini, oyster, portabella and crimini. Canvas awnings shade the produce, and on tables in the forefront sit huge wheels of parmigiano-reggiano. Scanning the vegetables, my eyes become transfixed on slender green artichokes with veins of a violet tones running throughout. The lengthy, fibrous stems of the 'chokes appear so vibrant and pulpy and their shapes so natural, I would rather paint a watercolor of them then to eat them. The celery too has this same rich green quality, with hardy leafy stocks that make their California counterparts seem leggy and watered down. Perhaps this is a better growing climate or could it be the volcanic soil? Dad decides to buy *due banana*: "It's important to keep fresh fruit in our diet when we travel," he reminds me, as he reaches out to grab the two bananas. His actions are met by the wagging finger of the produce vendor who firmly scolds him: "No Touch!" "No Touch!" As Dad waits for the vender to pick out two bananas, he nervously fumbles for change from his pocket. We pay the vendor and the two of us slink away, slightly embarrassed to be so easily identified as *turisti Americani*—guilty as charged.

By 9:00 A.M., the Milano Monday work morning is in full swing. Impeccably-dressed business people stride quickly and purposefully about us. Commuters on bicycles whiz by fully clad in suits and dresses, ringing the functional bells of their handlebars, forewarning pedestrians to jump aside. Not a single helmet can be spotted among the well coifed biking crowd. What a difference from the recreational riders of my rural California. Wearing micro fiber clothing, helmeted and gloved, we ride hunched over and sweating for a long endurance "workout." The Milanese ride their bikes right up on the narrow sidewalks. We jump aside and watch in amazement as they adeptly maneuver around us, gliding through pedestrian and vehicle traffic. Other commuters catch the trolley, the bus and the subway. "Look how efficient the downtown parking is!" Excitedly, Dad points out the numerous parking spaces set aside to accommodate mopeds, bicycles and small European cars. "And do you notice we haven't seen one SUV, van or jacked-up monster pickup truck since we got here?!" he delights. I nod in agreement and feel myself becoming incredibly envious of this walking and biking downtown culture. While Dad is mesmerized by the parking efficiency and modes of transportation, I continue to be distracted by the beautiful and svelte, olive-skinned men and women who move about this city. It's not just their natural good looks; it's this healthy glow and their upright postures that impress me. I have never seen such a well-dressed, trim and vital bunch of people before in my life. I feel that I have fallen into some vortex—a parallel universe—where perhaps all conditions might be perfect: the climate, the air, the affluence. It occurs to me that some of this may be due to the fact that Milano is considered the haute couture capital of Europe. I remember reading a statistic, some years ago, that over 1,000 models live in the downtown area.

The hair styles of the Milanese women are incredibly chic and the sleek monochromatic garments that drape their bodies look expensive. Suddenly, I have a burning desire to find a hair stylist who can dye my graying crown and give me a stunning, cosmopolitan cut. I'm ready to replace my practical, floral, travel skirt and sensible, flat walking shoes for clothing that make me feel like a hip city sophisticate instead of a country peasant girl. We notice almost every woman we pass sports the latest in severely pointed heels, something I do not envy. "They're ridiculous!" Dad laughs, as the heels clack to and fro about us. Later, a woman striding ahead of us gets her sharp heel caught in a sidewalk grate. She quickly stoops down, liberates the heel from between its rungs, slips the cruel shoe back on her foot and, as cool as a cucumber, glides away.

The pace of the bustling downtown increases well into the morning, and by midday we have explored some great neighborhoods and arrive back at the Piazza del Duomo. Hordes of people—locals and tourists alike—hang about the spacious piazza and chat. A cluster of about 20 Chinese people are gathered around a tour guide as they listen to the history of the cathedral. Dad and I exchange smirks, happy about our decision to travel independently without a tour group. The piazza is lined with cafes serving "take away" lunches, specifically little sandwiches called "pannini". Catering to the faster paced business crowd, Milano's version of fast food looks quite wholesome. Fresh baked breads, prosciutto, salami, cheeses and ripe tomatoes are some of the ingredients that are displayed within the glass-enclosed counters of the cafes. I spot a McDonald's and a Burger King wedged within the European architecture across the square, but no long queues exist outside their doors. "Let's get some pannini for lunch," Dad suggests, both of our stomachs growling by now. We quickly line up behind a lunch crowd inside a café and point to flat seeded buns, prosciutto & provolone. Our waiter creates an unpretentious sandwich including tomato and fresh sprigs of arugula which he then toasts between an iron press. Later, as we eat, I detect an infusion of olive oil which blends the distinct flavors into one complimentary culinary treat. For a second time today, Dad mentions the pride taken by our waiter. "He didn't just put the sandwich together and hand it to us. Did you notice the way he twisted the paper wrapping with a lot of flair, before presenting the pannini on the counter to us?" "It was all about presentation!" Dad enthuses. It's true. Our waiter may just as well have been presenting us with a flaming dessert or lobster tails.

Our room at the Hotel Speronari serves as a quiet refuge in the afternoon and by 6:00 pm we are back out on the streets seeking our first sit down meal. Dad warned me that he can't eat later than 6:30 in the evening, which could be a challenge in a country whose restaurant doors may not open for dinner until 7:00 or 7:30. We find an unpretentious, family-run place, located at the end of a short lane not far from our hotel. The oil cloth tables and plastic flower arrangements may not be the most elegant, but the *vino della casa* is great after a full day of pounding the cobbled streets. The *contorni* we order are simply *due insalate miste*: two mixed, greens salads. They are served with a carafe of olive oil and vinegar, which turns out to be the only way salad dressing is served to us throughout our travels in Italy and we love it. What makes this seemingly simple salad work so well is not only the freshness of the greens, but the quality of the olive oil and vinegar, requiring no other seasonings (although the salad often comes with fresh sprigs of arugula.) We had agreed early on that we would try to eat regional specialties during our travels in Italy—and in Milano that means *risotto Milanese* (rice with lots of saffron.) We also select a tomato *gnocchi* and wash it all down with our ½ litro of *vino della casa*. I note that none of the food we have had today is overly-salted or over-sugared. It is fresh, natural and without all the cheese that usually accompanies the Americanized-version of Italian cuisine.

It's been a full day. Dad is downstairs paying the hotel bill so we don't have to deal with it in the morning. We plan to rise early in order to catch the subway to the train station followed by a five hour trip to Venice. I am glad we planned as well as we did this past year. I can already feel the stresses of independent travel, particularly the transportation logistics and the language barrier. I'm relying on Dad pretty heavily, as I have no idea yet what I am doing. Dad's always thinking ahead: let's swing by the subway this afternoon to verify departure times. Let's pay our bills tonight, so we can slip right out of the hotel first thing in the morning. I learned a great deal from Dad about travel planning this past year as he purchased maps of the major cities of Italy, figuring the proximity of train stations, airports, and subways to the historic downtown centers. We chose hotels located within ½ mile walking distance to train depots and pre-purchased rail passes. We decided early on to travel light and settled on backpacks instead of rolling luggage. Friends had warned us that conventional luggage was more difficult to navigate than packs when it comes to jumping on and off crowded trains, managing the uneven terrain of cobbled streets and scaling three and four flights of the narrow steps of a European hotel.

This past year, Dad and I were regaled by seasoned travelers with numerous accounts of pickpockets, gangs of thieves who disguise themselves as business men, and women and children con artists who work in teams. One traveler recounted the incident of an elderly couple staying at a four-star hotel on a busy, fashion, "walking" street of Rome. Dressed in expensive clothing and gold jewelry the two were mugged immediately outside their hotel one evening. Dad assures me that a little street smarts and common sense go a long way for safe travel. He insists we find our hotel before dark when we first arrive to a new destination encumbered with our backpacks. Furthermore, neither of us wears jewelry (except our plastic watches) and we've tried our best not to look like tourists. We don't wear tourist khaki or tennis shoes and Dad delighted in his purchase of a green, wool beret cap, which makes him look like a distinguished, elderly Italian gentleman. We only packed what our airline carrier allowed in weight for carry-on luggage: Dad weighing in at a Spartan eight pounds and myself just under the limit of 12. To lessen my load, instead of bringing an entire guide book, I ripped out pages specific only to our destinations and organized them in a small zip lock baggie. I was left with a bit of extra space in my pack, which is good because I found myself dashing off to a department store this afternoon to buy a stretchy black cotton skirt, which already makes me feel a better fit in the Milano street scene.

After only one day in Italy, it is poignant the differences I am already sensing between my upbringing in the U.S. and a European culture. I question if this culture is more highly evolved and rich in its layers simply because there are more visible signs of history from which to draw. Certainly the European architecture must have some affect on the psyche and imagination of its people in a way that the big windowless box architecture of American suburbia could never quite deliver. My beginnings as a child in Seattle, Washington, with our backyard of narrow alleyways and the great walking neighborhoods, may come as close to a European influence as I have experienced: but this didn't last long. By the time I was seven, our family—my parents, three sisters and I—left our relatives in Seattle and moved to a suburb in California. Just two years later we were living in a small desert town not far from the Mexican border of Arizona and in another two years were back in California, again. Working in the field of computer science made Dad highly marketable, so he could easily transport our family to new locales; in retrospect I believe his decisions to relocate were based in part on a yearning to experience new horizons.

As a child, I too became swept away by new adventures. In the Arizona desert, my imagination was fed by the sight of coyotes, roadrunners, jackrabbits and odd looking arachnids and insects. When our family traveled to the nearby Mexican border town, I grew giddy with excitement knowing we were crossing into a different country. As hot and miserable as the desert could become, I loved poking around the abandoned, mining towns. When my family took hikes through dry river beds loaded with granite, I became a rock hound, stashing pieces of turquoise, quartz crystal, amethyst and tiger-striped agates into my pockets. I think it must have been during these years in the desert that the wanderlust truly started to take hold of me.

In six days, Dad and I will attempt to take a bus to Cuorgne, the small village and home of my Italian ancestors. Located in the foothills of the Alps, Cuorgne is not far from this very room in which I now write. A few elders we passed on the street today reminded me of my Italian grandparents: proud, reserved, modest and neat in their attire, the women of that generation always wearing skirts or a dress, nylons and pumps and the men in slacks and jackets. Today, I feel as though I may have stolen a peek into my grandparents' past. I wonder if Dad has too been visited by nostalgia.

Dad has returned to our room, after paying the bill for our lodging. Our bags are packed to allow time for an early morning cappuccino stop and a ½ mile walk to the Milano subway. As much as I have enjoyed my first Italian city, I am excited to move on and see what lies ahead. Transportation is about to take a dramatic shift as we leave the bustling metropolis of Milano for the vehicle-free islands of Venezia.

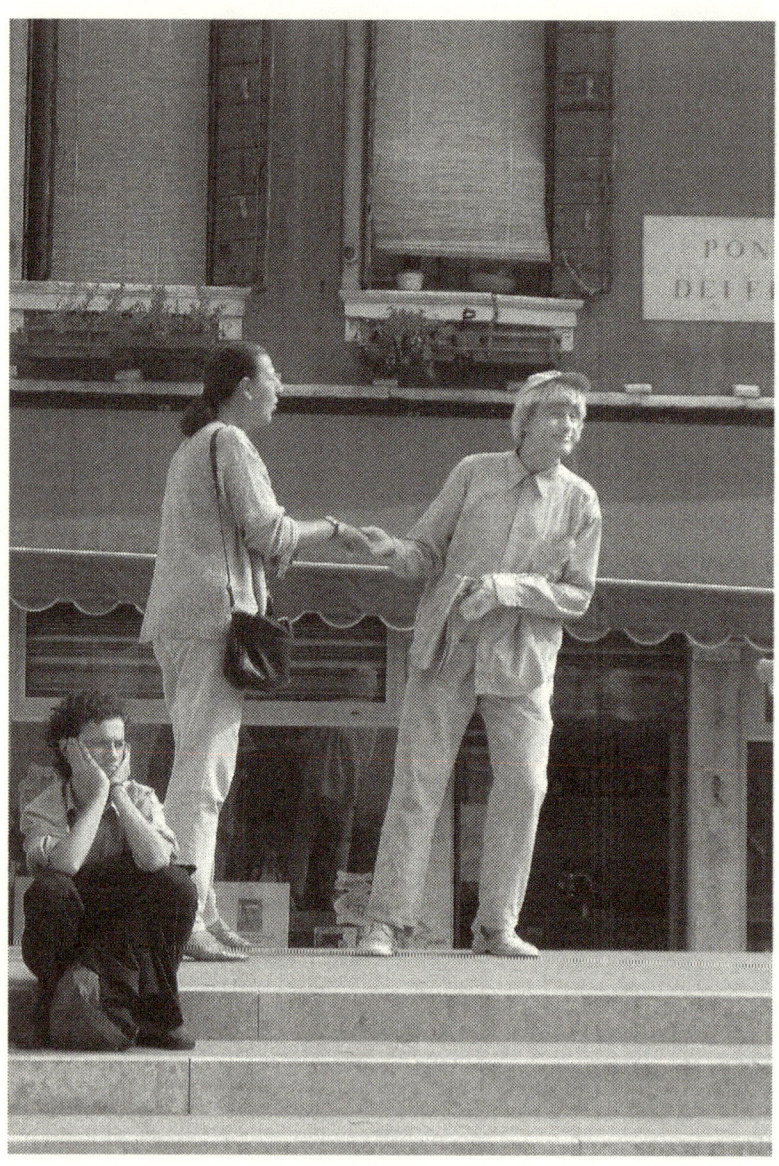

Venezia

Venezia

28 Settembre

To reach Venice this morning we board Tren-Italia at Milano's Stazione Centrale, a immaculate grand station boasting the immense fascist architecture of the Mussolini era. Headed due east, our train rambles for three hours through open country dotted by occasional villages. We pass time chatting with two Aussie travelers, as well as a young backpacker who is returning to Leeds after six months on the road. He smells like he's been six months traveling. The more talkative of the two Australian fellows tells me that Dad and I can pass for locals, which pleases me. His traveling companion, whose eyes remain obscured behind a pair of black shades, mentions to me that he will be in Venice for four nights. "Maybe I'll run into you" he suggests. "Probably not" I think to myself as I glance over to Dad and then back to the dark glasses.

As the train chugs closer to our destination, we pass through urban sprawl, refineries and smoke stacks until we leave the mainland altogether, crossing a causeway that takes us over the water to Venice. We have reached the end of the line and I can feel my heart pounding as if I am about to enter another world, like stepping into the Emerald City of Oz. Emerging from the train depot, immediately we know we're in tourist country, as backpack-laden travelers and piles of luggage fill the steps that lead down from the station. The scene before us is surreal—a movie set of gondolas and water taxis known as *vaporetti* glide along the Grand Canal. Arched bridges and candy cane striped mooring posts emerge from the water near the banks. There are no vehicles or motorbikes in sight and people are dressed casually, in striking contrast to Milano's week-day business attire. Meandering day trippers buy food and souvenirs at kiosks that line the *fondamenta*—which we later find out is the term for an avenue that runs alongside a canal. I draw in a deep breath of the salty sea air and relax as the moisture permeates my pores. Tourists dine at canal-side cafes, seated on awning-covered second story decks. We navigate our way through a melee of people until we reach the Ponte Dei Scalzi bridge that arches over the Grand Canal. By the time we have trekked over the bridge and away from the train station, the crowds thin considerably and I am able to pause and take stock of our unusual surroundings. A meandering hodgepodge of decaying buildings in pastel hues, this place is an artist's haven—a feast for the eyes. If you like the distressed, weathered look, come to Venice (before it sinks!)

Making our way through the Santa Croce neighborhood we serpentine into a cobbled maze of alleyways lined with two and three-story brick and stucco apartments that are wedged immediately beside the next. I see no trees, lawns or gardens on our jaunt to the hotel; instead, this appears to be an island covered in stucco, brick and cobbled stone all within a matrix of canals. An occasional brick passageway darts off into another alleyway that seems to disappear into nowhere. I am beginning to wonder how we can possibly stay oriented when it's impossible to see off into the distance within this jumble. Dad stops to ponder the map, already puzzled. He manages to get us back on course, and a number of wrong turns later, we locate the Hotel Dalla Mora—our digs for the next three nights. The modest, one-star *albergo* located at the end of a short alleyway, sits at the bend of a narrow canal. A young, friendly blue-eyed Italian man in the lobby points us to our room located on the ground floor. Cozy and narrow, the room has a big, shuttered window with a sitting ledge that looks out on the bend in the canal. Across the canal sit distressed-brick apartments that are accented by wrought iron balconies and window boxes brimming with geraniums. The Hotel Dalla Mora has the added feature of being run by a non-English speaking Italian family and all of this keeps us in a *non-tourist* state of mind.

We quickly unpack, anxious to hit the maze of alleyways and explore our unique surroundings. We discover that the Dalla Mora is located near a long stretch of wide alley—a thorough-fare by Venetian standards. The alleyway is a tourist hub of sorts, offering a number of appealing restaurants and several great looking gelateria. Sandwich boards advertise dishes of fresh fish and pasta and we decide to return here later for dinner. Before long, we fall into a circuitous maze that eventually opens up into an enchanting, rambling neighborhood of brick and terra-cotta tiled dwellings. Stairways lead up to small terraces and courtyards reveal an occasional stone Madonna perched upon a pedestal or a winged lion protecting an iron gate. Small arched bridges provide foot paths over a grid of narrow canals. I could ramble and skip through this for hours seduced by the angles and the pink brick that reflects back within the lapping patchwork of water. It is quiet here. There is no sound of motors. It is a seductive meditation.

The relaxed pace and fishy scent of the lagoon keep trigger-ing memories of the eight years that I lived in the California coastal communities of Santa Cruz. During my teens, I began frequenting the beach communities—just over the mountain pass from the Santa Clara Valley in which my family lived. After one semester of college, I dropped out, packed my bags and moved with my boyfriend to an affordable rental near the beach. Santa Cruz and her surrounding seaside towns were drop-dead beautiful. I loved the coastal air, the walking streets of the downtown, funky little shops with names like Bodacious Begonia, and the relaxed beaches and scenic drives. In the early 1970's, the inhabitants of Santa Cruz were predominantly a mix of retired people, seasonal vacationers and college students, while nature lovers like me were beginning to creep over from Silicon Valley. In the years to come, my new back yard filled up with artists, musicians, pot growers, horse back riders, surfers, transients, young entrepreneurs and Vietnam War vets, to name a few. The general community seemed peaceful and tolerant of people who were seeking new and alternative ways of living. It felt like home.

Each summer Santa Cruz ballooned to three times its size with mostly day-trippers, not unlike what I imagine Venetians experience much of the year. To remain living near the ocean, I held a series of mundane—but steady—jobs that did not exactly translate to a career track. As the years flew by, unfortunately my wages did not keep up with the increasing cost of living. Then, there was the slight problem of having put off college for eight years and a growing uncertainty of what direction to take next. I eventually returned to Silicon Valley, where, by day, I worked for a small computer programming company and, by night, sat through mind-numbing accounting and programming classes. It was the culture shock, however, that really got to me—for now I was back in a megalopolis of ugly suburbs, bumper-to-bumper traffic, strip malls and fast food joints. I felt suffocated and lonely, as by this time, my family and past friends had relocated elsewhere. I lasted only two years before my mea-

ger belongings were once again packed headed north to the small, rural town of Ukiah, where I would settle near my parents and a sister.

"Claudia! I can't believe it! How did we end up over here?" Dad jars me from my daydreams as he shakes his head at the map, looking thoroughly baffled. "It's a hodge podge!" he exclaims. "And the street names—Jesus! They change with every block and none of them seem to match what's on the map." Instead of entering the Emerald City, I'm beginning to think we have fallen down Alice's Rabbit Hole. Half-trusting the map, we reorient ourselves then continue through the maze until the alleyways abruptly end and open up onto an expansive body of water, what looks like a canal or inlet. A wide walkway—a *fondamenta*—follows the canal and appears to go on for several miles. Along the *fondamenta*, umbrella-shaded tables sit outside several cafes in preparation for evening patrons. Vaporetti and larger vessels travel along the canal and few pedestrians seem to tread this stretch of the island. We duck into an old, sea-weathered church where we find respite within the long shadows of the late afternoon sun. Faded Renaissance frescoes cover the entire walls and cracked ceilings, and a musty smell permeates our surroundings. When a middle-aged woman enters and kneels at a wooden pew, we leave her alone and continue our trek outside along the *fondamenta*. Across the waterway, we begin to spot several stark-white marble facades of palaces butted right up to the water's edge. The facades are flanked with faux Corinthian columns and adorned with flamboyant naked and scantily-clad figures that cavort gaily atop the peaked eaves. I have read that over a hundred of these palaces were built along Venice's grand canals between the 12th and 18th Centuries, at a time when the city was a formidable power of commerce and trade. The splashy facades now linger within this tourist lagoon—a lasting reminder of a conspicuous consumption that accompanied the wealth of a previous era.

Brick warehouses, that were at one time used to store supplies shipped from the mainland, reside along the *fondamenta*. We enter one that is functioning as an artist's showroom. Dark and cavernous inside, the only color comes from bold acrylic strokes that are splattered across large white canvases hanging from the brick walls. "They look like someone's post-apocalyptic nightmare," I tell Dad after we're safely outside again. "They're ugly!" Dad is more direct and equally turned off by the cold quality of art. Then it occurs to me that the abstract composition of the pictures resembles the menacing smokestacks of the refineries residing just beyond the Venice causeway. Briefly jolted from my magical illusion of Venice, I face back in the direction of the belching stacks that lie off in the distance.

"We had better turn back if we want get to the Dalla Mora before dusk," Dad wisely suggests. We retrace our steps along the *fondamenta* and zigzag back into the interior maze through a completely different neighborhood until we reach a small hub of tourist shops. I slow my pace to examine the huge hams and prosciutto that hang from metal hooks in the windows of a delicatessen. Shops filled with fine lace doilies, tablecloths, Mardi Gras masks, blown glassware and framed paintings all beckon *turisti* to come inside and spend, spend, spend. I wonder where the locals buy their supplies around here. I haven't seen anything substantial in our wanderings today, such as a produce stand or grocery stores. Perhaps the Venetians commute by train to the mainland or shop in neighborhoods we have not yet discovered to buy their goods. I would love to linger in this quiet business hub a bit longer, but Dad insists we press on, then successfully navigates our way back to the Dalla Mora before dark.

After hot showers, we follow our noses to the area we spotted earlier where the scents of garlic and fish now inundate the neighborhood. We find an inviting *osteria* and order a gnocchi dish with shrimp and a fresh pasta in a crab sauce. We can't see the crab—no big obvious chunks—but the flavor is distinctly of crab blended with garlic and herbs. We take turns digging and scraping the tiny morsels of shrimp from their delicate shells before finally popping them in our mouths. *"Molto Squisito!"* I try out the words I found in my phrase book earlier today. Our meals are brothy and delicious without relying on heavy creams or rich cheese sauces. The portions are reasonable, which seem to be about half the size of what is dished out to us in the good ole U.S.A. We have our usual *insalta mista* and wash it all down with a ½ litro of vino della rossa.

"We wandered way off into the Dorsoduro District this afternoon" back in our room, Dad points the area out to me on his map of Venice. My travel notes tell me this neighborhood is also referred to as *the tail of the fish*. Studying the map I can see now that the many tiny islands that make up Venice form the shape of a fish and that the Grand Canal cuts a wide jagged swath right through the center. The broad canal along which we strolled this afternoon turned out to be the Canale Della Giudecca, which appears to be about three times the size of the Grand Canal. And the dwellings and palaces that appeared across the canal were on the island of Giudecca. By the looks of the map, I realize I will probably remain hopelessly disoriented for the next three days, so I'll leave the navigating to Dad.

As the night grows pitch dark, a gondolier glides just outside our window, so close I have eye contact with him as I cross the linoleum floor on my way to the bathroom. Rowing through the watery night, I can hear him as he serenades his passengers with a folksy tune. Later, as I drift in and out of sleep, another gondola passes, this time the singing accompanied by a raucous accordion.

29 Settembre

Bright and early this morning we stop for our first cappucino and Brioche (we're up to two coffee stops a day now) then hit the cobbled maze in an attempt to find *Piazza San Marco* where the highly-visited St. Marks Basilica and the Doge's Palaces are located. I'd like to get this "must see!" out of the way so that we can relax for the remainder of our stay in Venice. Despite my efforts last night to painstakingly chart the most direct—albeit circuitous—route to St. Marks Square, we soon discover my time would have been better spent picking my nose. We're not two minutes into the maze this morning before street names we don't recognize appear out of nowhere and twists and turns arrive so quickly I discard my makeshift map altogether. Instead, we blindly fall in with a stream of pedestrians until we notice signs that read Piazza San Marco and simply head in the general direction.

Our route through the brick jungle this morning is dank and dark and not particularly pretty, like yesterday's wanderings. We arrive at St. Marks Square, over an hour later, foot sore, frustrated and disappointed by what we find: a spacious, treeless stone piazza already filled with groups of tourists. To add to the commotion, actors and extras dressed as peasants and cardinals of the Renaissance era mill about half-bored, as directors and a film crew prepare to shoot a scene. The splendiferous, onion-domed St. Marks Basilica appears more forlorn than regal, as it resides above this flea-market-like atmosphere. The marble façade of the basilica is a hodge-podge of architectural features and a mishmash of patterns not unlike the crazy streets upon which we have just trod. It's easy to read Dad's anxious expression as he studies the queues of tourists lined up outside the Doge's Palace. Instead of insisting we visit the historic treasures housed within, I take Dad from his angst and suggest we exit this Renaissance scene altogether. "We're outta here!" he rejoices, as we flee the piazza in search of our next cappuccino.

Following the *fondamenta* along the Grand Canal, I stop briefly next to a six-story high building to shove my sweater into my pack. Suddenly, a loud thud startles me, as a heavy bucket hits the pavement, splattering black streaks of tar across my legs and skirt. The alarming sound of Dad screaming, tells me he too has been doused. Shaken, we both stare up from where the bucket fell and observe an intent Italian man perched on the rooftop. Gripping onto a heavy rope, he is attempting to lower five remaining, heavy buckets to the street below. Concentrating on his primitive mechanics, he does not so much as flinch at the near death-by-tar experience he has inflicted on us. "You could have KILLED US!" Dad shouts up to the man, like a true Italian. We dash from the scene to avoid further incident, when an Italian woman zips alongside us, screaming something up in the air, her arms flailing in wild gesticulation. We have no idea what she is saying or even whose side she has taken, so I simply flash an appreciative grin and scramble with Dad to the nearest espresso bar. On a postcard to a friend, I scribble: *Falling buckets of tar is one peril Rick Steves failed to mention in his guide book!* (in reference to the popular travel guru.)

We spend the remainder of our morning poking around the Museum of Modern Art, the Gallerie dell'Accademia and exploring the surrounding neighborhoods. We assume there must be a school of art in the vicinity, as evidenced by students perched on nearby arched bridges with sketch pads and pencils in hand. The exquisite detail of the Byzantine and Renaissance architecture in this area inspires even me to draw—something in which I have only recently dabbled. Dad encourages me to stop at one of the art supply stores where I purchase several colored pencils. I fantasize in detail about the scene I would draw—delicate, swirling lines to suggest the archways, facades and domes against alternating patches of mustard, pink and muted green—the colors of my pencils and the palate of Venice. I place my artist's tools in my Rick Steve's day pack and wonder if they will ever see the light of day during our whirlwind trip through Italy.

Seated on the ledge of our hotel window, I scrub the tar off my legs with warm soapy water and let the sun beat down on my back. Mid-day is especially peaceful in our neighborhood and I enjoy the slight lapping sound of the canal. The gondoliers don't come by during the day. An occasional row boat of local kids or teens may pass, briefly breaking the absolute silence. I take time to peruse our Italian phrase book in preparation for our next outing. *We are still struggling with the language barrier and I have been finding that contrary to what I have been told about all Europeans speaking the English language, most locals we have encountered seem to speak little of it. I think I would have fared better—at the train depots and the restaurants—had I rehearsed some phrases beforehand. We've been surviving by a few simple words and gestures alone. In the months leading up to this trip, Dad and I took some Italian language classes, listened to tapes, practiced gender agreements, conjugated verbs and rehearsed imaginary conversations. Now, all this study and preparation seems mostly academic as we are paralyzed, speechless, by each question we are asked or direction we are given. One of the Aussies on the train yesterday assured me my tongue will begin to loosen by the second week. I hope he's right. He added that it helps that we both look Italian.*

This afternoon my next communications challenge comes soon enough. In search of a much-needed *birra* (beer) we wend our way from the Dalla Mora to *Campo di San Toma*, a neighborhood square frequented by local families. A few mothers are pushing baby buggies, a handful of children play about the square and some elderly gentlemen and women are seated at tables, *al fresco*. Several cafes seem more geared to tourists, with long cafeteria style tables set outside providing enough seating for big groups. We avoid these establishments and instead find a small bar set off on its own. Visiting the cafes frequented by locals also means we have to work more diligently at using our sketchy Italian language skills. Ordering *due birra* isn't too difficult; however, communicating that we wish to be seated outside doesn't come as easily for me. After some confusion on the waiter's part, I blurt out the words: *al fresco?* and he seats us at a wobbly umbrella-shaded table, close to other patrons. Only minutes into our pints of cold beer, Dad spills part of his, splashing the nylon-clad legs of a proper little 'ole Italian lady seated at the table beside us. Dad apologizes to her using the English language, but her expression is not one of understanding or forgiveness. Instead, she strikes me as being a local who has possibly grown weary of sharing her town with tourists. I forget about trying to conceal my tourist status and quaff a hefty swig of the Becks Beer, secretly thanking the Germans for the much needed libation. Before long, a group of school kids stroll over, drop their packs and seat themselves at a table. Ordering a round of espresso, they proceed to engage in lively conversation. I'm not sure if this scene is typical of how most Venetian kids spend their after school hours, but I'm impressed nonetheless at how sophisticated it all appears in contrast to my own adolescent after-school activities. By the time I was 15, my friends and I were frequenting the drive-through fast food chains. "Three cheese-burgers, two large fries, an order of onion rings and three choco-late shakes" we shouted our order into the mouth of the giant metal clown. Whizzing by the drive-through window to exchange money for grease-spotted bags of food, with cache of sugar, salt and fat firmly secured, we headed down the hormonal highway of life, our transaction requiring little more than yelling words into the microphone of a clown. I can't help but contem-plate the differences in cultural environments as I observe these polite Venetian kids tipping back the delicate white demitasse cups with their fingers as they continue to chat.

We enjoy the spacious feel of Campo San Toma this after-noon. The campo is flanked by three-story sea-weathered apart-ments that are accented with teal and evergreen shutters and small iron balconies. Eroded patches of stucco pockmark the exterior walls and expose a layer of brick beneath. Signs of flooding are evidenced by several feet of faded, exposed brick at the street level. I remember one of the Aussies had mentioned that many of the interiors in Venice (anything on the second floor and higher, that is) can be really quite elegant. It's hard to envision this, as I study the dank, sea-weathered exteriors before me. I have a feeling the Aussie must have been referring to the interiors of elegant mansions, which I can be sure will not be included on our self-guided itinerary. Dad poses beneath the brim of his green beret, as I snap a photo of him holding the ½ empty pint of *birra* beneath the awning of the café table.

I spend time in the evenings reading a paperback and writing my impressions in my journal, as the sound of music and party-ing emanates from somewhere off in the distance. This marsh-land of tiny islands is all beginning to feel rather claustrophobic, mysterious and moody to me—a never-ending hodgepodge of mazes, appearing to cater more to tourists than to the 60,000 local residents. I didn't study up much on Venice, but once Dad and I had made the decision to add it to our itin-erary, reading fiction became great fun as we dove into the moody atmosphere of the islands. We both read "Aqua Alta" by Donna Leon, a crime novel that takes place during the flooding season. We followed her protagonist, Commissario Guido Brunetti of the Venice Police, into upper story apartments and palace interiors, through cobbled streets swollen with the "high water", sloshing our way with him in knee high rubber boots across wooden planks set about the city. Another book I read "Vaporetto" by Robert Girardi, was altogether surreal in its full use of the lagoon setting, providing a great back drop to this tale of an insomniac and his plunge into the supernatural. Taking place mostly by night, within bars and dank alleyways, involv-ing a mysterious woman and otherworldly characters, with noc-turnal feedings of stray cats and references to the cemetery island of San Michele, I could hardly wait to see if Venice would possibly live up to all this pretense. "And then some" I note in my journal at the end of our second day in the cobbled jungle.

30 Settembre

We are surrounded by bright orange and blue washing machines of spinning laundry in a *lavenderia* this morning. I think I have been transported back to the 1970's, to the television studio set of "Laugh-In." Two small TVs recessed in the walls blare out the Italian news. A British man and his son just left the building, while a German couple enters and appears already to be struggling with the confusing operating instructions posted near the door. Dad, on the other hand, is clearly in his element as he seems to enjoy cracking the case of the baffling operating instructions. He flits about between the coin machine, the posted operating instructions and the washing machines, until triumphant I witness our clothing churning amongst a sudsy sea of bright washers. Could a morning in Venice get any better than this, I chuckle to myself, as I finish writing in my daily journal. I pick up the "The Worldwide Diary" a laundry-mat journal of sorts, added to each day by fellow travelers. Entries are scribbled in Italian, English, Chinese, German, French and Russian. One of the travelers writes that their stay at the Hotel Florida was great and that the panorama of Venice from St. Marks Bell Tower is not-to-be-missed. I cringe as I reflect on Dad and myself scurrying yesterday like cockroaches away from St. Marks Square, clueless that we had just missed the best view of Venice. Another entry from a young girl reads: *This is the nicest laundry mat we have ever been in!*

I think maybe my tongue is beginning to loosen. This morning I successfully asked the man at the front desk of our hotel for directions to the *lavendaria*. Impressed by my one complete Italian sentence, he proceeded in great detail to explain something incomprehensible to this here *gringa*. Nonetheless, he sent us off in the correct general direction and Dad managed to find our way with the map. We seem to survive to a degree by interpreting gestures from helpful locals, picking out a few key words and by gut instinct. It helps if you don't mind getting lost quite a bit. It's a hell of a good work out! I can see where it would be fun to stay awhile longer at the Dalla Mora. The family who runs the hotel is extremely friendly and cheerfully appreciative of our attempts to communicate. Although we never stay for the breakfasts that are provided—because frequenting coffee bars is much more fun—we received some of the Dalla Mora's personal laundry soap for our jaunt to the *lavendaria* this morning. I'm beginning to feel a bit like a seasoned traveler.

While Dad is in charge of laundry mat problem solving and transportation issues, I'm in charge of our daily excursions. This can be a daunting task, as I fumble through the ripped out pages of travel books I packed along. I look for sights that might appeal to both of us, while integrating a new walking route each day to check out the various neighborhoods. This afternoon, I suggest we visit the Santa Maria Gloriosa (St. Mary of the Friars) *a 13th century church housing masterpieces of Venetian Renaissance art.* After the requisite zigzagging through alleyways and tunnels, we enter a spacious cobbled square where a quaint, carnival-like atmosphere is unfolding. Beneath a grand, stone cathedral, a handful of tourists and locals mill about. A mime sprayed from head to toe in silver dungarees and work shirt uses a silver cell phone as his prop to parody passersby. I think his use of the cell phone is brilliant, since everyone in Italy seems to own one. They use them on the trains, in the streets, and some while riding their motorbikes. Again, my illusion of Venice is briefly interrupted when the silver mime breaks character to converse with this pony-tailed, flamboyant director and his small camera crew. An elderly black, blind accordion player, seated on a stool in the middle of the square, appears to be part of the filming as well, whether he is aware of it or not. When we approach the steps of the Renaissance cathedral we enter into an ethereal world. Unlike the dark interior of Milano's Duomo with its narrow, gothic, stained-glass windows, Santa Maria Gloriosa is well lighted by circular windows of mottled light-green glass. Inside is an impressive collection of statues, alters and sarcophagi, crafted with the finest quality marbles and gold. We spend the better part of an hour admiring the masterful art housed beneath one roof. I had noted Rick Steve's recommendation that his favorite way to see art in Italy is "in situ" and now I can understand why.

We leave the Renaissance scene at the *campo* and leisurely stroll to the north side of Santa Croce where we pick up *due pannini*. A series of shallow stairs flanking the Grand Canal serve as our rest stop. Moored boats bob rhythmically in the canal and marble steps of a nearby palace disappear altogether into the murky lagoon. It seems surreal—otherworldly—as I watch a modern-day water taxi zip down the canal, while trying to imagine what the moldy steps of this ancient palace must look like from beneath. After lunch, we discover the greatest hidden gardens and quietly cloistered courtyards that lie behind iron gates of grand brick homes. A whiff of marijuana overtakes us as we notice two young men with backpacks nonchalantly smoking at the dead end of an alleyway. We slow down our pace and continue our walking meditation through the quiet labyrinth. We have not seen a vehicle in three days now—no cars, no trucks and no bikes. The alleyways are filled with pedestrians only. Push-carts are used for hauling garbage, building materials, supplies—basically everything—back and forth to boats that are docked at the canals. I notice residents place one, small plastic bag of garbage in the alleyways immediately outside their apartments. In the early morning the bags are retrieved, loaded onto push carts, then hauled away by boat. We have also noticed what I refer to as the "pedestrian version of peak traffic hours." Streams of locals zigzag quickly through the alleyways between about 7:00 and 8:00 am, all heading for work we suspect, possibly to commute to the mainland by train. It seems oddly quiet as they serpentine purposefully through the maze, an unusual inertia accompanying their mass movement. Following the pedestrian rush there is be a brief period when the foot traffic abates altogether. Shortly thereafter, backpack laden groups of children, often accompanied by parents, navigate through the alleyways to school. Again, the foot traffic lets up and the maze becomes still. "It's the oddest phenomenon" I remark to Dad. "People traffic hours instead of vehicle traffic hours." It all appears somewhat comical and surreal when played out within the decaying medieval labyrinth.

We enjoy a phenomenal last evening meal at *Antica Osteria*. Lured inside by a great looking menu, a young Italian woman seats us at a white-linen draped table. The interior of the café is typical Venetian with shiny, exposed copper pipes lining low ceilings. American Jazz is being played and we are the only ones here at 6:30 PM. This place may cater to locals, for the moment our young waitress discovers we speak little Italian, she retreats to the kitchen and another waitress replaces her. The dish of marinated squid with dandelion greens is *fantastico* and the mussels and clams in a marinara sauce *molto squisito!* We take full advantage of being in Italy during the height of mushroom harvesting season and order the fresh fagliatteri pasta with Ceps mushrooms. "Ceps" Dad explains—or *Boletus Edulus*—are wild mushrooms prized by the Italians. They are common in the Piedmont region of Northern Italy, the home of our ancestors. He describes to me how his parents carried the custom of mushroom gathering with them to the U.S. *"They gathered mushrooms along the Teanaway River near our home in Cle Elum,*

Washington" he recounts. *"Then for a treat, Ma would simply sauté them—freshly gathered—in butter and onions. Delicious!"* Dad savors every bite of the pasta, impressed by its freshness and flavor. He tells me it is the food we have been eating during this trip that more than anything triggers memories of his childhood.

After our meal, I try out a new phrase on our Italian waitress: *"Complimenti al cuoco!* To which she immediately corrects me, insisting that I repeat the phrase—not two—but three times: *"kwo-ko, kwo-ko, kwo-ko"* I respond like a trained seal, until she is satisfied that I have correctly pronounced "compliments to the chef". Not only do some of the locals we encounter insist we learn the proper inflection of their regional dialect, a number of them—we notice they are usually around college age—go to great lengths to insist we speak no English whatsoever. I'm beginning to wonder if this effort is a reaction to the many foreigners who visit and overtake the Italian countryside with their own languages. At last, our waitress praises me: *Brava! Perfetto! Bene!* Having finally met her stamp of approval, we exit the osteria, fully sedated by our excellent meal.

This evening we trek over the Ponte Dei Scalzi bridge toward the train station. We'll be five hours riding the rail tomorrow so to avoid delay or mishap, we make sure to confirm our departure time and reserve seats in advance. Often, the railways that connect the larger hubs fill to capacity with commuters, so we have learned to reserve seats when traveling to the bigger cities. While Dad has become adept at determining the timeline schedule and departure platforms, I am becoming proficient at conversing in Italian with the ticket counter clerk. It hasn't taken long in our travels together to quickly find our roles as we work in tandem.

From the train station, we stumble into the lively Cannaregio District. Music reverberates from cafes, while crowds of young party-goers and tourists wander the trendy streets. *So this is where it's all been happening at night and without me!,* I reflect to myself, thinking how much fun this would have been about twenty years earlier. In the dark of the evening I can make out a neighborhood full of tall stone apartment buildings, which I would love to explore. This must be the old Jewish ghetto I have read about. I sense Dad is ready to meander back, so we order a scoop of gelato, then join a small crowd that is gathering around a street artist who adeptly uses the edge of a piece of charcoal to create a canal scene of Venice. We stroll along the *fondamenta*, where I notice a long dinner table of about 15 men donned in skull caps, dining *al fresco* near the water's edge. The night has grown pitch black by now and a cool evening mist is settling over Venice. We follow the *fondamenta* back to the Ponte Dei Scalzi bridge, and take the familiar twists and turns in the alley-ways until we reach the Dalla Mora. Dad uses the old brass key to unlock the door to our room for the last time and inside we ready our bags for an early morning departure to Turin. Located in the Piedmont Region of northwestern Italy, we will attempt an excursion into the foothills of the Alps … to the small village of our ancestors.

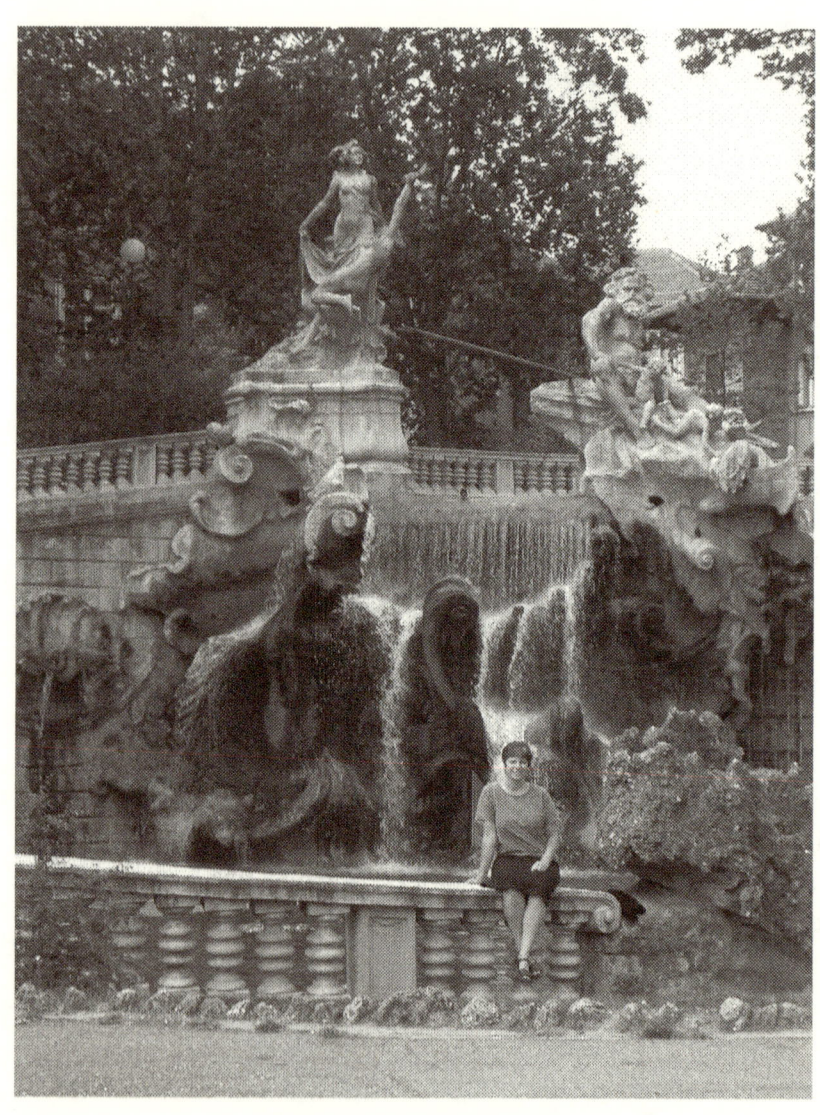

Torino—Along the River Po

Torino

1 Ottobre

We leave the sinking city behind and settle in for a five hour journey that will take us back across northern Italy, beyond Milan to the industrial hub of Turin, *Torino* to the Italians. Unlike Venice, Torino is not on most people's itineraries as a tourist destination. For us, it will serve as a base camp of sorts as we attempt to visit the small village of Cuornge. Our train rolls over the causeway from Venice, back onto the mainland and past the refineries of belching smokestacks. With the eyes of voyeurs, we watch for signs of other people's lives as the train cuts so close to backyards we see children's toys strewn about and laundry hanging on lines beneath windowsills. Discarded tires and rusted auto parts create heaps of unsightly rubble near the train tracks. Soon the signs of habitation cease altogether and we reach another long stretch of countryside.

It feels good to be back on the train. With as much walking as we have put in, the train gives me some down time to regain my bearings and feel a bit of separation from my intrepid companion. Dad and I don't talk much on these long stretches and I notice it irritates him somewhat when I spend my time journaling rather than being fully engaged in the countryside beyond our windows. He doesn't want to miss a thing and he doesn't want me to either. It wasn't until I turned 38 that I truly got to know Dad well. It happened during a time in my life when one event changed the course of my future. One sentence from your doctor and your entire world—as well as everyone in your sphere—changes overnight. "What beautiful weather we had today" my doctor's opening line cues me that I'm in big trouble. Obviously she isn't delivering the good news that my biopsy proved negative. I help her out with her next line: "DO I HAVE CANCER??" shocked, the words escape my lips, all too quickly. "Yes, you have cancer" she confirms lucidly. My mind slowly rises above my body, where it can safely observe these two individuals—like players in a script—having this incredible conversation, and one that certainly couldn't involve me—not with words like CANCER and MALIGNANT. My doctor is speaking rapidly now like she's sucked helium. Words and factoids are spewing from her lips in a jargon foreign to my ears. A few of the words stand out, however, that I DO recognize and understand: MASTECTOMY, CHEMOTHERAPY, HORMONE THERAPY. "Expect this next year to be stressful, filled with doctors, surgery, treatment." … "Do you need some Kleenex?" "Can I give you a ride home?" I can't breathe. I drive myself down the street to my sister Wendy's house. When I enter, she's complaining about a minor car incident that day—a fender bender. "Well, I can top that!" I interject recklessly, "I have breast cancer!" "You're going to be ok" she immediately assures me. It's all too surreal. Wendy is more somber later when she realizes that I might loose a breast, undergo chemotherapy and what about my chances of survival. I don't sleep one wink that night—nor does anyone in my family— and I had a great excuse to call in sick to work the next day: "I won't be coming in. I have breast cancer."

Yet, this crisis—this sudden facing of my mortality—somehow gave me permission to put my personal needs first. I felt compelled to face myself and my fears, to dive into the confusing, mysterious abyss of who I really am with all my scars and faults and hopes; and what I might do differently if given a second chance. That year I slowed down my pace both at my demanding job and in my social life. I learned about relaxation techniques, visualization and simply began considering new ways to exist in this hectic world. I distanced myself from my supportive and well-meaning boyfriend, as I started to attend to my own soul searching and healing. In retrospect, I was beginning a long journey inward. With my bald head, like the Buddah, I retreated to my cave just as often as possible.

Fortunately, by this time in my life I was living near family members, had a support group of friends and held a good job with excellent health benefits. Facing cancer can be a frightening and lonely experience; it was my Dad who took it upon himself to become my confident and personal advocate. He diligently researched breast cancer and later accompanied me to San Francisco for chemotherapy treatments. It was during these long stretches stuck in the car together that I truly got to know Dad well. He recounted tales of the year he took a hiatus from college to hitchhike with a buddy across the U.S. I pressed him for information about the lives of my grandparents and immigrant great-grandparents and listened intently to stories about the two years that he and my mother lived in Manama, Bahrain. As I relax on this train, in good health and over a decade later, I question whether Dad and I would have even considered traveling to Italy together had it not been for the disease that flung us head-on into each other's worlds. I study his face now that remains mesmerized by the Italian countryside. What a far cry this is from our days of journeying to San Francisco for the toxic chemotherapy. Knowing what we have come through makes this long overdue trip that much better.

Five hours have passed quickly since we left Venice. The Alps rise majestically off in the distance as our train inches closer to Torino. I peruse the pages I ripped earlier from my travel guide to see what's in store. "Industrial, "grand wide avenues of Baroque architecture", the home of the Fiat", "excellent gelato and chocolate", "progressive", the "slow food movement." As our train rolls through ugly, outlying, industrial sprawl, I mentally gear up for another bustling city and for our next train station challenge. *So far each station has been full of commotion, particularly the Malpenza station in Milano. I realized there would be stress and confusion navigating our way through a foreign country, but nothing like what we encountered that first evening at the Malpenza Station. We backtracked up and down stairways several times before we finally—20 minutes later—emerged upon the platform for the commuter express that transported us to the downtown area.* Again, the moment we disembark at the Torino station, pandemonium reigns. The station is packed with people and we spend a good deal of time trying to determine which of the numerous offices or kiosks manages the bus vs. train vs. hotel information. We need to book a room and are especially interested in finding a bus that will take us to Cuornge tomorrow. Using my sketchy language skills, we discover there are no modes of transportation available to the village of Cuornge short of renting a car, and since neither of us wants to hassle a car rental, suddenly the trip to our ancestors' village is aborted. This leaves us with two nights in a destination I would not have chosen—downtown Torino—"Not exactly Paris," I grimace to myself.

Despite our initial confusion at the train station, we are both impressed by the ease of using the Tourist Information (T.I.) kiosk for locating a hotel. The attendant readily pulls up a number of hotel options on the computer screen, we select a place in the downtown area and she reserves a room for two nights at the Hotel Nazionale. And what a deal it is—a three-star hotel at 55 Euro per night for two. With packs, we head out from the station and follow a wide boulevard that is bustling and noisy with vehicle and foot traffic. Trolleys, automobiles, vespas, pedestrians and the strong fumes of diesel engines tell us we're back in a thriving metropolis. Huge sections of the sidewalks and piazzas have been demolished and are under reconstruction, which we later find out is in preparation for the 2006 Winter Olympics.

Although the route on our map to the hotel seems direct, as usual, we get lost. Our confusion is in part due to the number of streets that are blocked off for renovation, causing detours around the downtown area. Frustrated and unable to find Via Roma, Dad blurts out to an approaching Italian man: "Via Roma?!" The young man is highly offended as he shouts back: "Next time you come to this country you should take lessons in Italian first!" His retort further confirms my suspicions that a movement may be under foot about tourists speaking the language of the land. The man soon admits that he speaks English fluently, but insists the three of us converse in Italian instead. We receive extremely complicated directions to Via Roma, manage to part ways with smiles, and find ourselves no closer to knowing our whereabouts than five minutes earlier.

We wade through more streets filled with rubble, until we find the Via Roma, a busy thoroughfare that leads to the grand, downtown square—the Piazza Castello. Wide, elegantly tiled sidewalks lead up to the piazza and overhead arched porticos go on for city blocks, which provide excellent shade from the sun. "Just think of the great walking you can do in the rainy season!" Dad delights at the functionality of the architecture. Numerous shops boast trendy and artistic window displays. Upscale coffee bars are attended by baristas dressed in starched, white shirts. The pace of the downtown is fast, upbeat and the people are many.

Off on a side street awaits the Hotel Nazionale—a gray, multi-storied, nondescript boxy high rise. The hotel touts itself as 3-star, but after we get inside, we suspect this rating may be a carry-over from its heyday, possibly 50 to 100 years ago. The concierge in the lobby is surly and doesn't crack a smile. Up the elevator to the third floor, we emerge and follow a cavernous, high-ceilinged stark white hallway accented by outdated lighting fixtures and a few small pictures hung unimaginatively at random.

Our room—located at the final bend of the vacuous hall—is huge, like a cave. Small twin beds, each with a metal gooseneck lamp placed at the headboard are overwhelmed by two-story high ceilings. Tiny, framed, still-life pictures of fruit get lost in the grand space above each bed. A desk, a chair, two armoires and a small, white refrigerator that sits on the carpet still leaves the room feeling immense. Walking across the room, with brute force, I jar open a large, shuttered window, letting in a loud cacophony of vehicle traffic from below. I notice we are afforded the visual sensation of a non-functioning cement foun-tain—a huge, ill-sculpted, half-nude lady in repose. Her muscu-lar torso looks less like a woman and more like a man with two peaches plopped on his chest. I check out our spacious bath-room and delight to discover a claw tooth tub—at last, a chance to soak my weary bones in hot water. Dad, on the other hand, is impressed by the amount of square footage we have just obtained for $55 Euro a night. "This is the best room yet!" he beams as he chooses a bed and starts to unpack.

Clanking within the bowels of the Hotel Nazionale, we see only one other couple during our two-day visit. My imagination gets the best of me as the movie "The Shining" comes to mind: the fright of finding oneself alone in an empty and isolated resort hotel during the off-season with no residents other than your own family member—who also happens to be a mad-man. When my bathwater doesn't heat up, Dad finds the manager who sends his henchman—a nervous, humble, good looking, muscular fellow—an aging Italian James Dean. I notice he sports a black and blue thumbnail, speaks no English and seems intimidated by us, or perhaps by the communication barrier. The trick to the hot water problem—James Dean signals to us—is to first allow the water run a good 15 minutes. Eventually, I get to relax in the almost-hot water for about three minutes before it turns tepid. After our first night, we commiserate about the squishy, springing mattresses. But for 55 Euro and centrally located, it's a decent room, so we stay on.

Our first night out in Torino I try a new approach with our waiter in my attempt to speak Italian. *Buona Sera! Parliamo un po l'italiano*, I let him know right off the bat that I only speak a little Italian. He is quite gracious and our meals turn out to be excellent. The most memorable item this evening, as simple as it may sound, is the fresh, home-made *grissini. Grissini* is the term for breadsticks which are traditionally served in a basket at almost every restaurant we visit in Italy. This grissini happens to be outstanding: not hard and store-bought, but freshly baked twists of warm, chewy dough. A fresh grilled salmon steak and *risotto di frutti di mare* (brothy rice with mussels and shrimp) makes for excellent fare and hardy sustenance. And sustenance we will need, for as my journal entry later notes: *"…. got lost again this evening walking in circles. I really like Torino though. I love the grand avenues of bookstores, bars and hip window displays. I like being in a city that doesn't cater to the tourist trade."* We remain lost almost our entire stay in Torino. The unfamiliar downtown area and pockets of neighborhoods and restaurants seem wide spread across a lot of terrain, so covering ground for us feels like a marathon. Even if we splurged and took a taxi, instead of pursuing everything by foot as we do, neither of us would know exactly where to direct the driver. This is a hell of an exercise regime we're on and it justifies our second gelato today. Dad orders a delicious, fresh *crema* (vanilla) and me a *nociolla* (hazelnut.)

2 Ottobre

Today we plan a rest day. I was happy to discover that the grand River Po slices through Torino with miles of meandering parkway following both sides of her banks. We decide to escape the bustling downtown and enjoy a picnic al fresco at the river. We've been eyeing the tantalizing food displayed in the delicatessen windows—petite torts and soufflés, whole baked succulent chickens—many dishes appearing to have an influence from nearby neighbor, France. At an off-the-beaten-track coffee bar, we stop for our requisite *due cappucini e Brioche*. I haven't exactly pinpointed what it is about the coffee in Italy, but I like it much better than its American counterpart. The coffee seems creamier, not as thin, and I appreciate that less milk and foam are used in the cappucino. The small ceramic cups serve probably no more than a real cup measure—a good shot, yet not so much to set the belly and nerves on edge. This limited portion gives us a great excuse to sit down to another serving later in the morning. I can see that coffee, food and gelato breaks are fast becoming the driving force of our daily wanderings.

Heading to Torino's east side, we cross a wide, arched bridge that spans the River Po. Exquisitely-sculpted, Romansque statues reside at either side of the many bridges that connect her banks. On the east side, we find ourselves in a neighborhood of affluent homes and estates peppered within tree-studded hillsides. Looking back across the river toward the downtown, I feel like I must be in Switzerland or Austria as the Alpine peaks create a magnificent backdrop to the city. The delis in this neighborhood are *fantastico*. We enter one that displays trays of marinated squid, fried zucchini, artichoke tortes, game hens, and many more dishes I don't recognize. For our picnic, we select a warm, crusty, zucchini torte and a succulent slice of juicy, tenderloin served with a delicate, dark gravy. The Saturday morning streets are quiet—free of weekday commuters. Along the greenbelt, we pass a few families with young children in tow. We take our time exploring the open, rolling, parkway, a real treat following the past days of navigating the closed-in configurations of Venice and Milan.

In the afternoon, we return to the Hotel Nazionale and don't emerge back into the streets until 6:00 PM. By this time, the Piazza Castello is swarming with people; groups stroll four and five abreast along the crowded wide walkways beneath the high porticos. Numerous bars with open doors are serving free *ciccheti*—small appetizers—similar to a pub crawl or happy hour. We have a hell of a time finding a decent restaurant that isn't packed on this Saturday night, so we spend a couple hours dashing about lost in the surrounding neighborhoods. Although I am famished, I long to slow down Dad's wicked pace so I can feast my eyes on the avenues upon avenues of tall Baroque buildings we have stumbled onto. Many of their upper stories are elegantly appointed with balconies held aloft by the sinewy marbled backs of men—the likeness of Atlas. We cover a good deal more ground before we find a place to dine, then spend the remainder of the evening cruising the trendy window displays of the downtown area. I notice a number of bookstores are selling Michael Moore's *Farenheit 911* in both the English and Italian languages. I had no idea how closely Europeans follow our politics and elections. Several times on this trip we've been asked by locals about our feelings toward President Bush. Adamantly, we both insist that we DID NOT and WILL NOT vote for Bush. *"Bush e molto male"* (mah-lay) becomes Dad's party line. The whole world is watching our superpower with the upcoming elections in November and I can feel the impact the U.S. has on other nations. I can feel it with each curious local who presses us for our opinions. Traveling as an American under the current administration and political climate makes me somewhat defensive and uneasy. Before we left the U.S., I half-joked with Dad about sewing small Canadian flags on our back packs to help soften our image.

Dad's reading a paperback by Lawrence Block this evening while I catch up on my journal. This afternoon I tried contacting a group of friends via the Internet, but due to my forgotten password, I had to abandon my efforts. These friends of mine are gathered today in Sundance, Utah, celebrating the ten year anniversary of a mountain climb we took together in Argentina. To fully explain, I must rewind to 1993, twelve years ago, to San Francisco. I suppose this is when the next big door in my life truly opened. It was during a routine visit with my oncologist, Dr. Kathleen Grant, when I learned about the mountain climb. The chemotherapy treatments by this time had ended and by all appearances my life was back to normal. But I didn't want normal anymore. I desired something much greater in my life and more meaningful than the mundane tasks afforded by my office job. Above all else, I felt an urgency to connect with other women who had experienced breast cancer and was compelled to give back in some way what I had learned from my experience. It was during this routine physical exam that Dr. Grant handed me a photograph of a beautiful snow capped mountain." Mt. Aconcagua—23,085 ft." I studied the caption typed across the picture. "I have a patient, Laura Evans." Dr. Grant began "She has been under my care for an advanced-stage breast cancer." Dr. Grant went on to explain that several years earlier, Laura had endured a bone marrow transplant and was confined to two months in an isolation chamber. Prior to her diagnosis of cancer, Laura—already an outdoor sports enthusiast—had become enthralled with mountain climbing. During her two months in isolation, she vowed if she ever emerged from that chamber alive she was going to climb another mountain. This time, however, she would climb with other breast cancer survivors, in an awareness-raising effort, as well as to offer inspiration and support to the millions of women and families struck by the disease. "You came to mind, Claudia, as one of my patients who might be interested in applying for the climb" Dr. Grant continued that day. "You always brought a positive energy during your office visits and I am of aware of how you exercised throughout your treatments. Your outspokenness and activism with breast cancer this past year, I think would be a great asset to this team". All this was true, I thought to myself as I considered the successful walkathon I had co-produced that year with Nancy, my friend and a fellow breast cancer survivor. Our efforts brought 150 participants, along with representatives from the local health community, together in our town park, as an awareness-raising and community support event. Shortly thereafter, Nancy and I formed the first support group in Ukiah, specifically geared to women with breast cancer and, free of charge. I had enthusiastically shared these endeavors with Dr. Grant and obviously she had taken note. Still, I was no mountain climber. Why would I be interested or even capable of scaling a 23,000 ft peak? "Laura tells me there will be a Trek Team" Dr. Grant went on to explain "a support team that will climb to base camp at 14,000 feet. This will open up the expedition for more women, not only those with high-altitude climbing experience." Now I was beginning to listen and by the time I got home from San Francisco that night my mind was reeling with visions of climbing a mountain with other women. As it turned out, I encouraged Nancy to apply as well and one month later we received a call from Laura that she wanted to meet with us. We met her in San Francisco during the weekend of the Race for the Cure. She queried us with a number of questions and shared her enthusiasm about her vision of the climb. Mt. Aconcagua, she told us, is one of the highest in the world, yet is less risky to scale than Everest and would not require the use of oxygen tanks. The expedition would be led by her friend, and world class mountain guide, Peter Whittaker, of Rainier Mountaineering, Inc. (RMI.) Laura by now had enlisted a team writer, a professional fundraising organization, and had created a board to oversee the project. "Expedition Inspiration" she beamed, was the name of her project.

As it turns out, Nancy and I were selected as the first two women to join Expedition Inspiration. From that point forward, we had 15 months to get in the best shape of our lives. Overnight, my concerns of a recurrence of cancer dissipated as this positive, exciting mountain climb came to the fore. I am certain there is a mind/body connection involved with our happiness and well being. As I contemplated the months ahead I could already feel my endorphins rejoicing, like a shot of morphine through my system. My daily life took on new meaning and lifted me far above the realm of the routine. Instructors at the community college invited me to speak in their classes about cancer and the climb. I wrote a series of articles for our college newspaper as the activities surrounding the mountain climb began to grab the attention of our community. Dad, himself an accomplished athlete, became Nancy and my self-appointed coach, encouraging us up the surrounding hillsides in our county and pressing us to increase our exercise regime with each passing month. That year, Laura recruited a total of 16 breast cancer survivors from across the U.S to be a part of our team, ranging in ages from 20 to 60. From a continent away, Mt. Aconcagua was about to become the centerpiece in the lives of the women, families and friends of Expedition Inspiration. We would touch the hearts of many people during those extraordinary months and our hiking boots were never far from our sides.

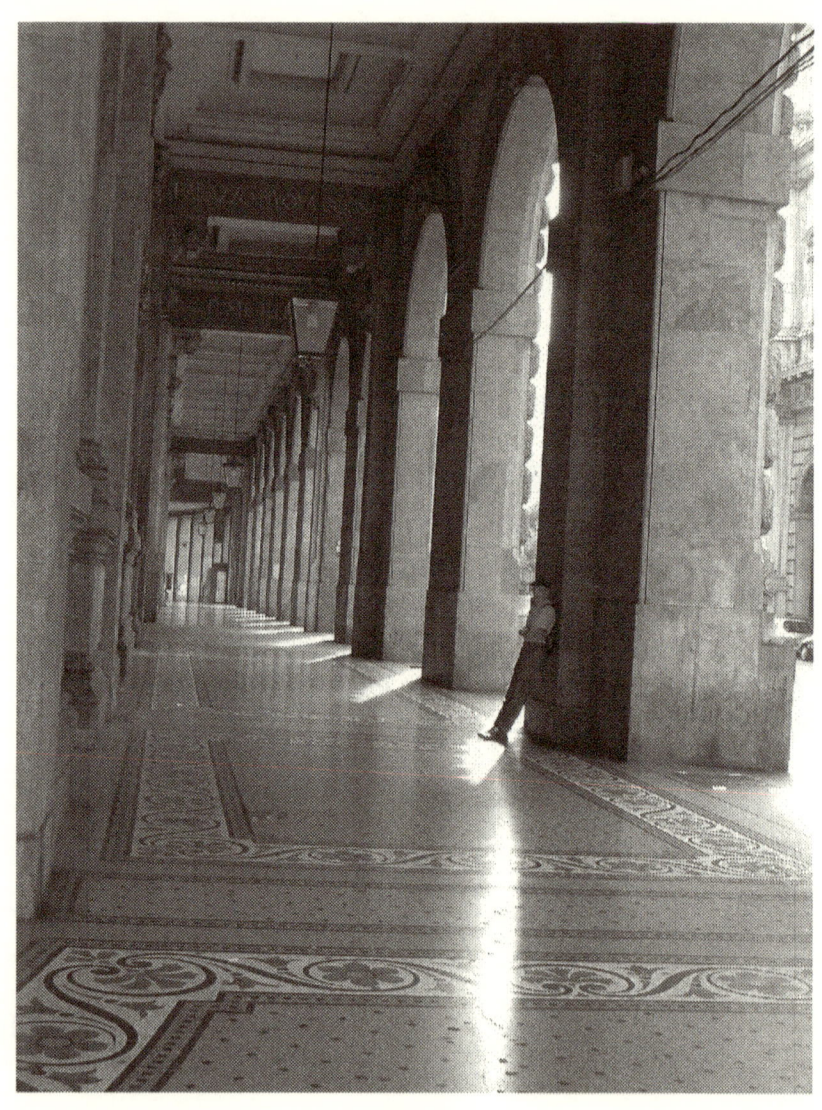

Genova

Genova

3 Ottobre

Arrivederci Torino! Our morning train is headed south toward the Mediterranean seaport town of Genoa, referred to by the Italians as Genova. At Genova we simply transfer to another train that will transport us along the Ligurian coastline to the tiny fishing village of Vernazza. Vernazza is one of five villages located on a remote stretch of the Mediterranean known as the Cinque Terra (or Five Villages.) We hope to enjoy a couple of days of sea air and relaxation in Vernazza, before moving on to the city of Florence.

With the outlying sprawl of Torino behind us, the train chugs into the Appenines Mountain Range. My travel notes tell me the Appenines begin near the Mediterranean at Genova, sprawling inland and then traversing down the center of the country like a spine well south into Italy's boot. As our train winds deeper into a dense, forested wonderland of mountains, I gaze out the window spellbound by this beauty that surrounds me. Villages of stone appear from within the trees, barely noticeable if not for a church steeple that indicates civilization. A castle rises from a ridge top. We enter a mountain tunnel and re-emerge to see another quaint village of stone and yet another castle. My blissful reverie is suddenly broken when a conservatively-dressed woman in our compartment asks if Dad and I are from the United States. She introduces herself and her teenaged son who are returning from a weekend of visiting relatives in Torino. *"Will you be stopping in Genova?"* she speaks with a thick

French lilt, typical of the Piedmont dialect. When I reply *no*, that we will be transferring on to Vernazza, she responds emphatically: *"that's a beetch!"* As with every Italian we have encountered on this trip, each is extremely proud of his or her own town and region and seems less than enthusiastic of all others. I wonder if this attitude is in part a carry over from the days when all regions of Italy were separate countries and that territorial pride is still deeply ingrained in the Italian people. Reminding me of a school teacher or travel guide, the woman begins to describe the great architecture of Genova. *"This is where you see the Genovesan style architecture: the layers of black and white marble on the cathedrals and palaces. This year Genova is also sponsoring a modern architectural show with structures erected throughout the city,"* she enthuses. Proudly, she informs us that the symbol of Genova—being a port-town—is the lantern or lighthouse and that the city is built on the hillsides like an arena reaching down to the sea. *"Genova is a beautiful city! You should not miss seeing it on your trip." We can help you buy a bus pass for the day."* She asks if we have a map with us, then proceeds to chart out a good route around the downtown and *porto antico* (old port) area.

By the time we are finished poring over the map, Dad and I are easily swayed and excited about delaying our arrival to Vernazza. I appreciate our good fortune of sitting next to the knowledgeable and assertive Genovesan woman. We have no guides on this trip—and dad is loathe to do a tour of any sort—so this woman's brief history of the area and her assistance comes as close to having a personal guide during our 20 day stay in Italy as we will get.

At the Genoa terminal, we check the departure times to Vernazza and discover we can catch a 5:00 PM, which should deliver us to the little fishing village by dusk. The Genovesan woman and her son stand in line with us and handle the bus pass transaction. Their assistance probably saves us 20 minutes of frustration trying to communicate with the clerk at the kiosk. Barely knowing the language is challenge enough; not knowing the bus system unique to a particular town is even more daunting. Bidding the kind woman and her son *mille grazie!* we check our packs at a baggage room at the station. Merging out onto the streets of the city we can feel a warm, sunny day in store, so we decide to forego our bus passes altogether, and begin walking instead toward the seaport.

As it turns out, we both love Genova. Unlike the flat, circuitous downtowns of this past week's wanderings, Genova is built upon rolling hillsides that lend a relaxed feel to it. The lush, tree-studded hillsides above the downtown and old port area in which we are now headed, are filled with homes and what could be palaces. A blast of sea air relaxes me immediately as I inhale a deep lung full of the soothing current. Trekking away from the station we follow Via Settembre, a wide avenue that leads us gradually upward. Romansque-style architecture is the setting for shops, businesses and cafes that we pass. Via Settembre peaks at the top of a hill, where we ramble for several blocks beneath covered porticos, treading across beautiful mustard and sienna patterned tiles. Heading abruptly downward toward the port, the cobbled streets narrow into a steep, vehicle-free, old charming *centro antico*. Rows of canvases set on easels display the work of local artists. Dad stops to examine a wooden cart packed with leafy bunches of Genovese basil. *"I have never seen basil so healthy!"* Dad leans over to inhale the pungent leaves, greatly impressed by the robust specimens. The produce vendor, dressed in velvet green Renaissance garb and leotards, keeps a watchful eye on Dad, and seems relieved when we move along. Across the lane, a mime poses like a marble Renaissance statue, sprayed head to toe in solid white. Her eyes are closed and her expression is solemn beneath a hooded toga. A copper-lacquered wreath of leaves forms a halo around her forehead. Her white-gloved left arm cradles a large hard-bound book, opened to its center. A few feet in front of the white column on which she stands, sits a copper-lacquered tip jar matching the halo on her head. "A classy mime" I think to myself, as Dad wanders over and empties his pockets of coin, dropping them in the copper container. Immediately the mime springs to life, as she mechanically, yet gracefully extends a delicate gloved hand high in the air producing a long feathered, fountain pen. With great aplomb and a generous smile she gestures for Dad to come sign his name in the register that remains cradled in her left arm. Dad gladly plays along and informs me later he signed the register *Vittorio Crosetti*. The mime quickly returns to her frozen stature, but not before giving me one big wink of an eye as I snap her photograph.

Continuing toward the port, we reach Duomo di San Lorenzo, an impressive, towering Romansque cathedral of the black and white striped marble design described to us by the Genovesan woman. Three magnificent arched doors to the cathedral are framed by elaborately-patterned columns of black and white spiraling marble. One perfectly twisted solid white column stands out in contrast to the rest: sculpted from the smooth, luscious Carrara marble it reminds me of a long, wide umbilical cord. I run my hand upward across its cool surface and am reminded that the fine Carrara marble is mined in the mountains south of here.

We reach the *porto antico* where our noses are greeted by smelly fish markets. Old brick buildings line the narrow streets accommodating gelaterias, cafes and tourist stalls. Window displays of fresh fish packed on mounds of ice boast lobster, squid, anchovies, mussels, clams, prawns and entire heads of swordfish, their swords positioned right in the line of the customer's vision perhaps for dramatic effect. We ramble onto a wide promenade that runs along a sea wall as the Mediterranean now spreads out before us. The warm sea air brings a relaxed pace to the pedestrians and the dress is casual. The seawall is lined with tall palm trees and the promenade is peppered with street venders. This is the first time on the trip I have noticed African people, so tall and lean and their skin so strikingly black it almost looks blue to me. The venders sell scarves, leather goods, cheap jackets and shirts. An old galleon—a likeness of *The Santa Maria*—rests in the harbor alongside a number of modern structures. One such structure looks like a huge round terrarium floating on the sea. I think it might be an aquarium, but it's hard to know since the guide book on Genova that Dad purchased back at the train station is a French version: he obviously missed the words on the front cover: *Genes—Images D'une ville*. I notice a large, open-air, platform or piazza of sorts that floats out on the harbor. A picture in *Genes—Images D'une ville* shows the floating piazza entirely lit up in the dark of night, with an audience seated before an orchestra underneath an open winged canopy rooftop. I wander out on a dock and lean over the rail to admire the crystalline, blue Mediterranean. Her water is so clear, I can watch schools of anchovies skirting over rocks, just beneath the water's surface. Facing back toward the city built on the hills, I see that indeed we are in an amphitheatre. Genova scoops downward from all three sides, like one half of a bowl to the sea. It's easy to understand why Italian people head for the Mediterranean to cool off during their vacations in August. And it's not hard to understand why our lady friend of Genova is so proud of her city. After several hours of meandering, we return back up into the hilly street sides above the *centro antico* and hoof it back to the station in time to board the 5:00 PM train to Vernazza.

Our train glides along what must be the most beautiful section of the globe I have ever traveled. This is where the Apennines Mountains dramatically meet the sea—so rugged and steep, it is a stretch of the coastline that remains underdeveloped. To the left of our compartment windows spread a range of steep, unfolding well-terraced mountainsides of vineyards and gardens. From within the mountains' creases, appear small clusters of stucco villages awash in muted tones of dusty rose, sienna, tea green and plum. To our right and for miles in the distance, rugged cliffs drop severely to the sea where they collide with long stretches of glimmering shoreline. Seaside towns we pass bear lyrical names like Camogli, Recco, Portofino and Rapallo. It is absolutely breathtaking, and I believe our 5:00 pm train departure out of Genova could not have been better timed, as the late afternoon sun bathes a calm Mediterranean sea in a brilliant canvas of pink and gold.

Dad is chatting with a young man from Milano who is seated in our compartment alongside his girlfriend. I notice he speaks English quite well. His girlfriend timidly tells me she speaks *l'inglese un po*—just a little. The young man boasts that he is treating her to a two day holiday in Monterossa, one of the five villages of the Cinque Terra. "Neither of us likes Venice" he declares. "Instead, we like to come to Monterossa for holiday." We learn that he lives with his parents in Milano, which continues to be (until one gets married) a very common and economic way to live in Italy. He holds a job that involves some travel to London and recently returned from a business trip to New York and California. He adores Starbuck's and would love to start each work day off with a *Grande Frappacino*. He loved being introduced to American waffles. He hates Los Angeles, as well as Sacramento and has no idea why a friend recommended Sacramento—let alone Sacramento's Old Town—as a *"must see!"* I giggle as I try to picture him striding the wooden planked walkways of the old frontier village wedged within the city sprawl, a far cry from the greatness of Rome. The kid doesn't stop talking the entire stretch of the ride. He loves New York City, enjoyed San Francisco, and doesn't understand why people would erect a roller coaster and boardwalk in Santa Cruz, thus destroying a perfectly beautiful shoreline. Not long into our conversation, a group of noisy women board the train. Their grand entrance grabs my attention, because heretofore—other than some cell phone noise pollution—the crowds have been relatively reserved. In fact, in the bustling streets of Milano and Torino, I noticed an unusual absence of talk among the passing pedestrians. It seemed that although the vehicle traffic could be noisy, the crowds overall appeared reserved. Now, as this boisterous group of women bustle by our seats, armed with shopping bags and luggage, I watch the young man from Milano grimace and proclaim under his breath: *"I hate old Italian ladies. They're from the South. The people from the south are SO NOISY."* He adds that he hates the Mexicans in California and Mexicans in general, yet is emphatic when he declares: *"Believe me—I am not a racist."* I can only imagine how all this is registering with Dad, who seems to be enjoying the exchange. When I mention to the kid that Naples is one of our destinations I notice he winces and responds with no comment. Our chatting has made time fly along this spectacular leg of our journey. The next stop on the train tracks is Monterosso, where we wave *arrivederci* to the young couple who now disembark. Five minutes later, exhausted from another day of considerable trekking, we arrive in Vernazza, the little fishing village tucked away in a spectacular fold in the mountains.

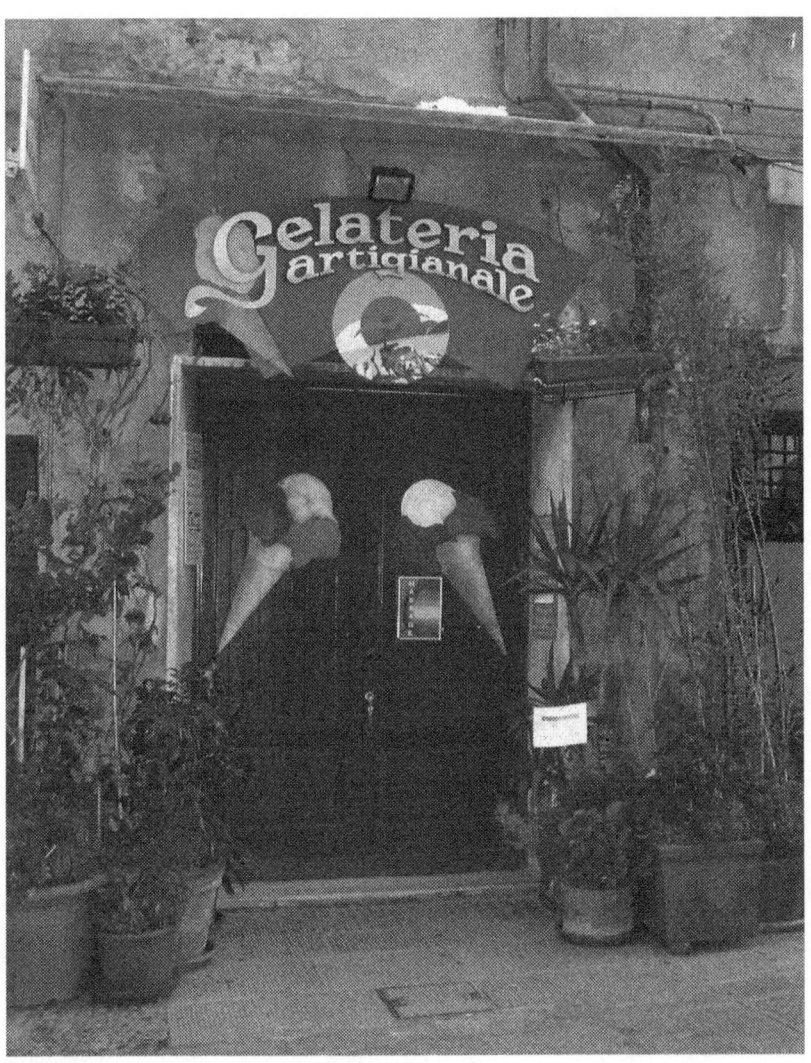

Vernazza

Vernazza

4 Ottobre

It is our second day in Vernazza. I relax for a spell in the afternoon shadows of the tree-shaded *piazzetta*, a small square located directly across from our pension. From where I sit on the far side of the square, I face back to a potted olive tree and a potted palm which accents the approach up the short steps. A black cat lolls beside me on the wooden bench we share. Healthy cats are a common sight in Vernazza. They bask about in the sun on rocks, within shops and restaurants, inside the hulls of small boats at the harbor, and among the many weathered nooks and crannies of this charming fishing village. By the healthy appearance of these satisfied felines, I suspect they receive some of the bounty of the sea and the scraps from restaurants that thrive here in response to the tourist invasion of recent years.

Our pension is located in the lower level of a three-story, mint-green, stucco apartment with tall, shuttered windows that looks out onto a cobbled street. We're one of many such residences located several blocks uphill from the train tracks. Although there are no hotels in Vernazza, a number of locals have turned their homes into vacation rentals and Anna Maria, our hostess, is one such enterprising local. A creek trickles about ten feet beneath a foot bridge just outside our pensione. It is quiet in this location of the hillsides, especially in the evening, save for a resident goose that wanders the creek side and honks occasionally night and day.

Vernazza is wedged in the crease between two steep, terraced mountainsides. The train tracks cut through tunnels in the mountains and right through the center of the village, several blocks downhill from the location of our pension. Periodically, throughout the day, we are startled by a thunderous boom and then we remember it's only the sounds of the train that has just cut through the tunneled cliffs and is preparing to stop at the depot. The only main drag in Vernazza is the Via Roma, a steep, cobbled street that descends below the train station all the way through the tiny town until it ends at a beautiful sheltered harbor. The Via Roma is lined with tall, colorful stucco apartments, homes and a small business district of sorts—a farmacia, two gelateria, a fish market, produce stands, some tourist shops, restaurants and the like. The working harbor is sheltered by dramatic cliffs and is the setting for a handful of modest restaurants, whose outdoor tables are shaded beneath colorful oversized umbrellas. By day, Vernazza's cliffside jumble of pastel dwellings are festooned with lines of laundry lending a gay, happy feel to the little fishing village. The high ridges above town are terraced with vineyards that overlook the Mediterranean. As I sit in the piazzetta within the sheltered folds of the mountainsides, I swear I have never in my life breathed air like this. It's as if I am in one immense, roofless arboretum where the moist sea air meets rich fertile soil.

Earlier today, I noticed a number of black and white photos hanging in the hallways of our pension, depicting past years of storms and flooding at Vernazza's harbor. I read in *Rick Steves Italy* that during the rainy months, the 500 local residents of Vernazza move to city apartments. Steves also mentions that wine production is not what it once was and that although locals still maintain family plots and continue to produce local wine, the younger generations have been choosing other, less physical, occupations. In fact, in the past two days I have noticed a number of the young locals waiting tables and working in tourist shops. There is no doubt Vernazza has become a tourist destination, geographically isolated that it may be. This is the most American tongues we've heard since first stepping foot in Italy. Last night at dinner, a bleached blonde and her friend seated at a table beside us wanted to strike up a conversation, but their harsh American accent felt grating to our nerves. In the past week, Dad and I have managed to surround our senses in this wonderful Italian bubble that neither of us is willing to burst. We have suspended from all forms of media, have not been barraged by billboards, telephone lines or golden arches, and have been swept away by the melodic rhythm of the Italian tongue. Comprehending almost nothing that the Italian people are saying, has somehow further enhanced our foreign bubble, and ability to suspend. Even while visiting the popular tourist destination of Venice, we found it easy to dodge the tourist areas and savor this foreign flavor to which we are both growing quite fond.

The residents of Vernazza seem to live amongst the tourists fairly peacefully and in fact thrive on them economically. Elders remain true to the evening *passeggiata* and children play alongside meandering *turisti* with little notice. When we first arrived to town last night tuckered out from pounding the streets of Genova, locals helped guide us to our pension. Foot-weary, and encumbered with our packs, we had hoofed it from the train depot, bustling downhill through a melee of strolling locals and tourists, until we reached the harbor below. Already apparently looking incredibly lost, I was delighted when three elderly gentlemen seated at a table outside a restaurant shouted out in their native tongue what I assumed meant *"what street we were looking for?"*

Beaming optimistically back at them, I responded: *"Fontana Vecchi!"* to which they signaled us back up from whence we came. Retracing our steps back up the Via Roma and past the train depot, another local man pointed us further up the road, until at last we found our pension. Rapping on the outside door of the building's first floor met with no response, so I poked around to the side of the pensione where I discovered a flight of stairs leading up to a third landing. While contemplating my next move, an elderly Italian woman leans out from a window of an adjacent apartment and starts shouting out some Italian words. From her body language and tone, I could sense she was friendly and assumed that she had gone through this ritual many times before. I was beginning to feel it was all simply a part of the rhythm of Vernazza. I smiled back to her and screamed *"Si!"* not knowing what else to do, then she gestured me to the 3rd floor landing which turned out to be Anna Maria's private residence. It was around 7:30pm by this time and when Anna Maria opened her door, I could see I had interrupted her evening meal. I introduced myself in Italian: *Buona Sera! Chiamo Claudia Crosetti. Ho una prenotazione per due notte.* Anna Maria, who seemed delighted to discover I spoke the language, responded cheerfully in a rapid succession of Italian phrases. I quickly learned that Anna Maria does not speak one lick of English and she in turn soon discovered I was unable to comprehend her words as well. Together, we hustled back down to street level where Dad waited patiently. Anna Maria showed us to our spacious, floor-tiled, spotlessly clean room and managed to pantomime a few house rules to us, most specifically about what not to discard in the toilet. Last night we fell asleep to the sound of the babbling brook just beneath our window, disturbed only occasionally by the honking of one resident goose.

Many hardy souls travel to the Cinque Terra to hike the cliff-side trails connecting the five villages along this remote stretch of the Mediterranean. These hikers are easy to identify as they emerge into Vernazza from the hills above, clad in boots, back-packs, trekking poles and sun hats. Earlier today, while we were down at the harbor, I noticed several groups of them trekking through town looking a bit peaked, perhaps in search of a liba-tion, a good meal or a refreshing dip in the sea. By noon today, a number of people were swimming in Vernazza's calm, scenic harbor. "I'd be out there too!" Dad announced to me as he eyed the swimmers in envy "but I didn't want to pack the extra ounce of weight just for one swim." Instead, we sat against sun-baked boulders and looked on as a group of hikers, gabbing in German, navigated slippery rocks. One of the women slipped into the water up to her knees despite the aid of her aluminum trekking poles. *As the pole released from her grip, my mind jogged back to the months leading up to the mountain climb. As Expedition Inspiration drew near, packages from sponsors began arriving to my apartment bearing gear—trekking poles, fleece jackets, thermal underwear, wool socks, climbing boots, backpacks, daypacks, a high altitude down sleeping bag and duffle bags of all sizes. Paul Delorey, the President of Jansport, manufactured our team merchandise, underwrote all team travel expenses and provided tents for the mountain. At a young age, Paul had lost an aunt to breast cancer and his heart remained closely aligned to our cause. Without hesitation, the women of E.I. embraced Paul's cheerful and supportive pres-ence and insisted he climb with our summit team. During prac-tice climbs and team gatherings, the women of Expedition Inspiration bonded easily as we divulged our personal stories and exchanged information about everything from complimen-tary treatments and ways to boost our immune systems to learn-*

*ing more about each others families and dreams. I noticed
immediately that all the women of our team shared a great love
of nature, as well as a desire to serve as activists in health care
or in our environment. I remember during my months of soul
searching, I promised myself one thing I would like to do more
of if given a second chance was to begin hiking again—something I had not done since the days of my youth. I had no idea at
that time that my wishes would come to me in the form of a
mountain climb in Argentina—and with soul sisters no less.*

I set down my pen and leave the piazzetta, crossing the street
to our pension. Dad has just finished hand washing a few clothes
and has hung them on the nylon line below our outside win-
dowsill. It is late afternoon and we decide to take our own little
trek up the dramatic cliffs that rise to the east of the village. We
climb past stucco apartments, terraced gardens, a fat cat eating
pasta from an open page of a newspaper and several groups of
hikers as we ascend the cliff sides. Continuing upward, the views
of the town and harbor below appear dramatic and sublime in the
low shadows of the late afternoon sun. At a lookout, we gaze
down at a church built into the mountainside just below us. We
visited this cathedral earlier today, welcomed by the waxy scent
of burning votive candles. Unlike the great duomos of the cities,
this church was designed with unpretentious, open-beamed ceilings, modest wooden pews and contains no marble statues or
windows of stained glass. What this simple church *does* have is a
fantastic setting. Facing toward the sea, the view from the tall,
clear-glass window of her quiet, simple interior was far more
uplifting to me than the cathedrals of marble and gold.

We reach the highest peak of the mountain trail where a well
cared-for cemetery overlooks the Mediterranean. Within tall

iron gates, perched upon a grassy knoll, rows of gravestones reside, many marked by black and white photographs portraying generations of families. An elegant, marble statue of Jesus rises above the headstones, his arms outstretched toward the sea. In the light of the sinking sun, it is truly a beautiful and moving sanctuary. I think we are alone, until Dad mentions afterwards that an elderly woman was weeping over one of the gravesites. We wonder how often she makes the arduous trek up from the village below and for how many years.

We decide not to take the stone path that traverses the terraced hillsides and instead, head back to Vernazza, like two barn-sour horses in search of dinner. Occasionally we pass hardy locals—some with babies and young children in tow—who commute by foot to and from town to outlying homes wedged within the mountainsides. We are equally impressed by the elderly who take their evening *passegiatta* up and down the Via Roma, undeterred by the cliffy cobbled terrain. Both evenings, we notice Anna Maria sitting with a woman friend at a bench in the piazzetta. Her friend knits while Anna Maria chats animatedly, both of them casually observing the parade of locals and tourists who pass them. Anna Maria always acknowledges us with a broad smile and a friendly wave of her hand as we emerge onto the street outside the pension. This evening, I see an Italian man is clowning around the bench where the two women sit. He is trying to grab their attention as he breaks into a ditty. Anna Maria and her friend respond in total disregard and shoo him away like an unwanted child.

For our last meal in Vernazza, we dine *al fresco*, at a harbor side café. Rather than a full dinner, we sit down for early appetizers to avoid the hassles of a busy tourist crowd at sunset. We order a focaccia appetizer and—upon the recommendation of our waiter—plate of *acciage fritta* (fresh anchovies.) The tender anchovies are breaded, pan fried, and served with ¼ wedges of fresh, local lemon. They are *molto squisito,* not-too-salty, and go perfectly with our *due birre* and an evening sunset.

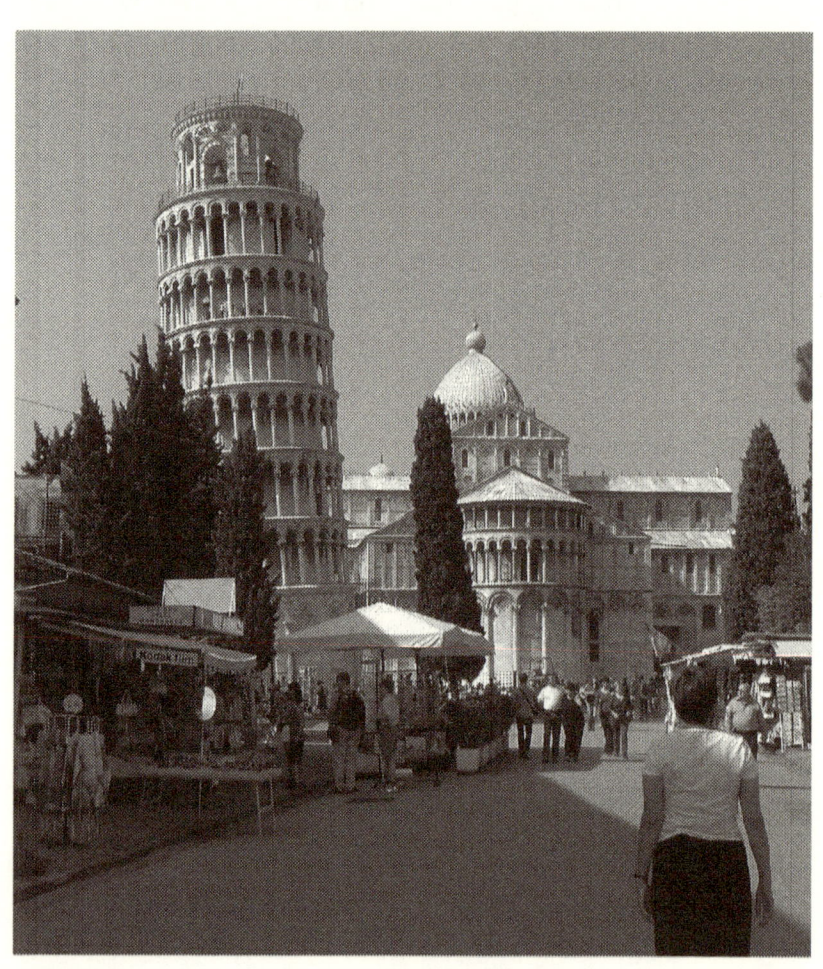

Pisa

Pisa

5 Ottobre

I adore vacations. And I'm finding that, like Dad, I too like to be on the move. Having chosen to live on my own for most of my adult life, I have found that solo living can be depressing at times, particularly in a house void of my now-deceased cat. Sharing vacations and waking each morning to a new horizon and to a travel companion brings me renewal and great joy. My elation is further buoyed by the awareness that I won't be working, cooking, cleaning, doing dishes, paying bills or making my bed for another two weeks. And so it is on this tenth day of our trip, that Dad and I zip our packs, sit down for a morning cappucino, trudge back up the Via Roma to the train depot and roll out of the tiny fishing village nestled in the crease of the mountains.

We are headed inland to Florence—called *Firenze* by the Italians—where we have booked ourselves for four nights. Our early morning train rumbles through more tunnels blasted in mountainsides and by small villages of the Mediterranean. We pass the seaside towns of Marina di Massa and Marina di Carrara, which I have read are popular destinations for holidaying Italians. To our east, we notice bald foothills of white marble that rise above the town of Marina di Carrara…. "the highest quality marble" my notes read "unrivaled in its texture and purity." The Carrara marble was used in Tuscany by masters such as Michelangelo as well as Brunelleschi in the building of Florence's cathedral. Until I came to Italy, I had no idea the variety or abundance of marble that exists in this country, nor have I seen it so widely used. We are surrounded by it daily: it flanks the exterior walls of cathedrals and bell towers, adorns the interiors of palaces and churches and is seen in the statues, fountains and monuments that visually enhance Italy's city streets. There is something about the oldness and permanence of our stone surroundings that deeply affects my psyche. This habitat is profoundly different from my environment in the America West where I live predominantly within a wooden framework of architecture. When I try to relate my impressions to Dad he reminds me that these stone buildings are not subject to fires, as is the case with wood. "These buildings survive from generation to generation" he muses. "They outlive us." While I consider this, Dad studies the map and proposes a divergence: "It shouldn't take long to get to Florence today. How about checking out one of the towns on en route and make it a lunch stop?" I mull over the idea, concerned it might take away from our time in Florence. Perusing the map I notice that our train stops at Lucca, a walled-in city full of Romansque churches and an old Roman ampitheatre. We also have easy access to Pisa. "How about Pisa?!" Dad interjects, while looking over my shoulder. "Alright, let's do it!" I surprise myself at how quickly I agree: I must be getting the hang of this spontaneous train travel. Pleased with our decision, Dad folds the map back neatly in his pack and twenty minutes later we are off the train and checking our bags at the Pisa station.

Immediately, we can tell Pisa has a small town feel, compared to Milano or Torino. The train depot is a modest size with only a few people milling about at this hour. We enjoy a leisurely stroll from the station around the southern edge of town as we intentionally take an indirect route to the leaning tower. Pisa is a university town with an open, easy feel. The busier streets are full of students commuting by bike. Sprawling neighborhoods of brown stone homes and apartments are thoughtfully broken up by tree-filled parks. The only area notably filled with *turisti* seems to be in the vicinity immediately surrounding the leaning tower.

The truly striking thing about the tower of Pisa may be the way in which we unknowingly approach her. To begin with, unlike many of Italy's grand cathedrals and bell towers which are cloistered within a maze of alleyways, Pisa's streets are more open and afford a distant vantage point. As we 'round a corner within the neighborhood of old, browned-stone buildings, the tower comes looming into sight, several blocks off in the distance. The tower's stark white marble exterior, angling downward at its impossible tilt, creates an almost comical illusion to the upright, brownstone buildings in our foreground. And for two people who had agreed months earlier that seeing this famous attraction was "no big deal", I find it amusing how quickly we pick up our stride, hypnotically drawn to the tower like a magnet, like a scene out of "Close Encounters of the Third Kind." In no time we cover several city blocks until we reach a promenade of kiosks that line the avenue leading up to the tower. I am distracted momentarily by my favorite tourist stall—the ones displaying aprons sold throughout Italy. A giant wedge of *parmigiana-reggiano* adorns one apron, the map of *Italia* another. My favorite, however, is the naked torso of David: from neck to knees, his well-sculpted, iconic figure covers the front of the apron, with his famous *pene* dead center to the garment. Dad scurries by and ignores me as I hold the garish souvenir up against my body. "Take my picture, Dad" I taunt him as he presses on toward the tower.

We circle the tower a few times and make a quick promenade around the grounds of the nearby Cathedral and Bapistry. Neither of us is interested in joining the queues of tour groups waiting to be herded inside. This means our visit to this *NOT TO BE MISSED!* tourist attraction lasts less than 25 minutes. "We're outta here!" Dad's jovial words match his buoyant step as we hit the cobbled streets in search of lunch. We avoid the blocks of tourist-filled restaurants near the leaning tower and wander a number of streets away until we find a restaurant with a good-looking menu that appears to attract a healthy local crowd. Since the front room of the *ristorante* is filled to occupancy, our hostess leads us to a pleasant back room filled with oil-cloth draped tables. An elderly Italian gentleman dressed in a suit is eating a slow, quiet meal accompanied by a ¼ litro of vino. Two gentlemen eat and chat quietly at the table beside him and three women are leaving just as we enter. We agree to be seated at the end of a table for eight which is currently unoccupied. While studying the menu, with beers already in hand, our waitress approaches and asks if we mind her seating a party of six alongside us. Politely we nod *"no problema!"* At first we are a bit uncomfortable at the prospect of sharing our lunch in close proximity to strangers, but this lunch turns out to be the most memorable of our entire trip. We don't understand a word the group is saying, but we enjoy being voyeurs—as well as a part of—this group of working Italians during their mid-day lunch break. The five business men (and one woman) are younger than the patrons at the other tables and end up finishing their delicious looking *pesto rigotti* more quickly than the rest of us. They seem to enjoy Dad and me as they smile and nod at our bold noble attempts to use the Italian language with our waitress. Our meals turn out to be as memorable as our company—a warm, creamy risotto with blended, soft, chunky, cooked asparagus throughout and thick, fresh spaghetti cooked *al dente* with steamed muscles and garlic. Our cheerful table-mates finish their meal with a quick round of espresso and bid us *arrivederci*. Satisfactorily sedated by the excellent food, we meander back to the depot to board the train that will take us to Firenze.

As our train rambles into the Tuscan countryside, Dad rarely averts his eyes from the scenic beauty and stone villas that begin to surround us. As much as I know he is truly enjoying this trip with me, I think he especially wished to have been on the mountain climb. He envied our seemingly exotic adventure and couldn't believe my good fortune of having fallen into a climbing expedition. At first Dad held out some small inkling of hope that perhaps there would be a slot for "a dad of a breast cancer survivor". But as each new woman—each breast cancer survivor—joined the E. I. team, it became clear that this was an exclusive group and a journey best shared from the sidelines. Besides, he didn't envy the criteria for joining our team— a previous diagnosis of breast cancer—no thanks. How well I remember those whirlwind months leading up to the mountain climb. Fundraising events were taking place in the cities of my teammates across the U.S., PBS had contracted to film a documentary, and Nancy and I were being featured in local newspaper articles and radio interviews.

By the time Expedition Inspiration departed the U.S. in January 1995 we were 43 strong: 17 breast cancer survivors, ten mountain guides and a nurse and three doctors who practiced in the field of cancer, one of whom was my own oncologist, Dr. Kathleen Grant. A film producer, camera crew, two professional photographers, Paul Delorey, our team writer, and Laura

Evan's husband, Roger, completed our team. The Summit Team departed the U.S. five days ahead of the Trek Team. It was esti-mated, by the time the Trek Team set foot on the trail, the Summit Team will have already reached Base Camp at 14,000 feet. The two teams would not actually unite physically until after the summit attempt was made. If all went as planned, the Summit Team would reach the 23,000 ft. peak and descend back to Base Camp the following day where at last we would reunite.

The Trek Team departed from various locations throughout the U.S. and converged in Buenos Aires where we spent a glori-ous day and two nights. We then flew across the country to Mendoza—a sprawling city situated at 2,000 feet in the foothills of the Andes Range not far from the Chilean border. Several days later, we were loaded on a bus that transported us into the beautiful Andes Mountains. Everyone was in great spirits and most of us were experiencing a certain amount of "performance anxiety" as the climb was at last upon us.

We were dropped off at a climbing lodge, referred to as the Hospidaje, located at 8,000 feet in the Andes. Here we repacked our gear, weeding out our street clothing, so that we were carry-ing only the essentials. On the day prior to our mountain jour-ney, a few of us got a sobering preview of the realities that lie ahead. We watched as a Dutch climber, who had fallen at 20,000 feet and spent a freezing night separated from his com-panion, was loaded into an ambulance. His pallor was bluish-white and he was suffering from frostbite and pneumonia. "He's obviously in shock" Dr. Grant observed, startled by both the physical and mental state of the man. She reminded us what a serious undertaking the expedition was. Dr Grant had the added stress of being one of our team doctors, responsible for overseeing any illnesses or injuries in the days to come. She seemed nervous about the dusty, hostile environment before us, particularly since she had a series of cataract surgeries, leaving her almost blind in one eye. Other members of our team were dealing with physical limitations: Patty suffered from chemo-induced full-body arthritis and Roberta was on double doses of Tamoxifin keeping her inundated with hot flashes. Personally, I worried about altitude sickness in general—headaches, nausea and any of the other climbing maladies that can set a climber back. I would be busy on this expedition and could not afford to grow ill. In addition to the physical climb itself, our team writer, Andrea Gabbard, had commissioned me to chronicle my daily impressions of the Trek Team, while she documented that of the Summit. I had 15 rolls of film I intended to shoot to use for slide shows and I had contracted to write articles for two periodicals upon my return. It helped that I was in the best shape of my life. I was going to need all the strength I could get.

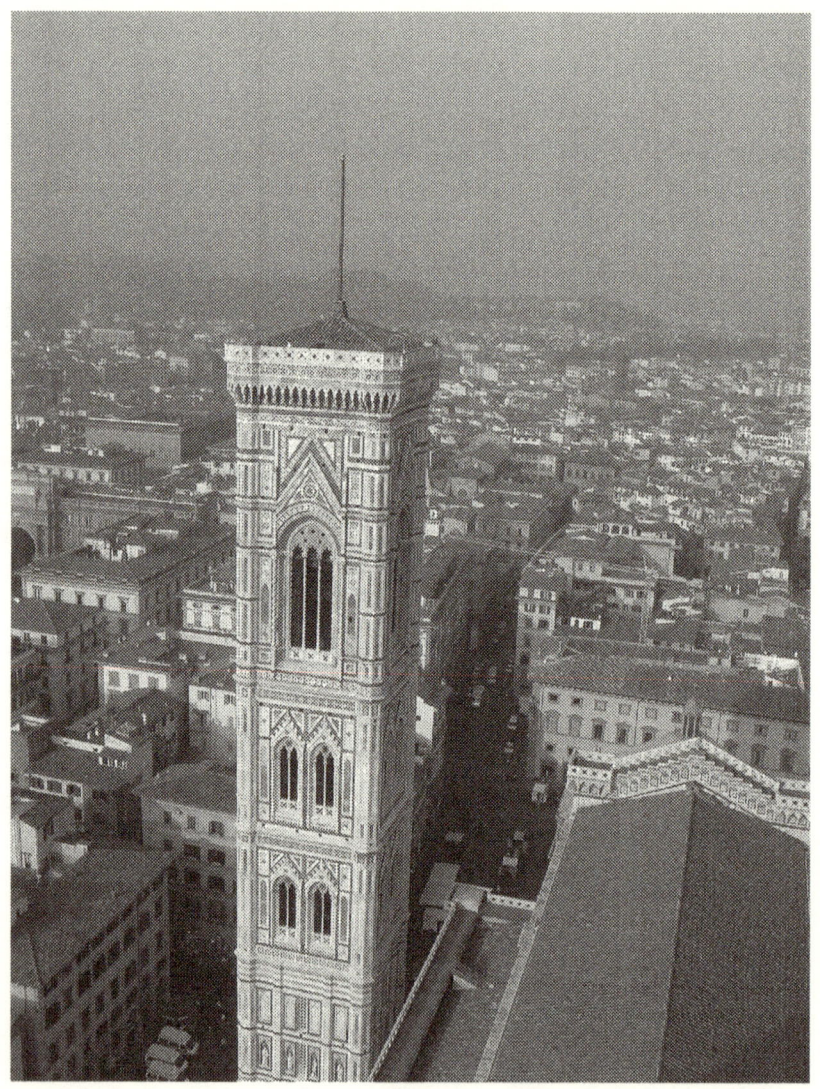

Firenze

Firenze

5 Ottobre

Of all the destinations listed on our itinerary, for me Florence held the greatest appeal. These past months I have been imagining myself meandering through an aesthetically pleasing, Renaissance city, an open air museum of architecture, marbled sculpture, grand piazzas and beautiful gardens. Glossy photos in travel books show a sea of terra-cotta tiled rooftops, churches filled with art, the Ponte Vecchio Bridge splendidly arching the Arno River and Florence's famous Duomo. My greatest concern has been how we can possibly fit it all into three-and-a-half days. So why then on a postcard to my sister, only Day One into Florence, does the greeting read: *Florence! Just another dirty Italian city!*

Because that's exactly how it appears to me as we emerge from the train station, where gobs of milling tourists and lingering locals fill the depot steps. Darting across a wide avenue, noisy with idling tour buses, honking automobiles and squirrelly motor bikes, we head directly for our hotel. Treading across the gritty Piazza di Santa Maria Novella, it's funny: the piazza doesn't look anything like the picture I remember from the tour book. Rubbish is strewn hither and yon and some homeless looking sorts loll about the unkempt grounds. The back alleyways leading to our hotel seem foreboding and narrow. The tall, dark, stone buildings feel especially bleak following the more rambling open cities of Genova and Pisa, not to mention the natural beauty of Vernazza.

Pensione Scoti—our refuge for the next four nights—is located on Via De Tornabuoni, a bustling street of high-end fashion stores. I feel frumpy with my backpack as I slink by Prada, Gucci, Versace and Louis Vuitton. Inside the shops, huge, plasma screens display ongoing footage of rail-thin models, full lips and high boots, accompanied by the piercing, monotone thumping of techno tunes. I do not even own an outfit that would allow me past the scrutiny of the impeccably dressed tall, black doorman, who stands frozen like a statue, barely averting his eyes as we pass.

Dad and I get an upper body work-out pushing open the 15 foot high steel doors that open to a grand foyer of the building where our pensione is located somewhere on the 2nd floor. On the opposite side of the foyer, we step inside a tiny elevator, which has a capacity for about three underweight people bearing no luggage. The elevator stops at the 2nd floor where we pivot our bodies, open an opposite door of the lift, manually shut the door behind us, cross another landing, ascend a short flight of stairs, and at last open another door where we find the delicate gold lettering that reads *Pensione Scoti*. Our room, overlooking a quaint courtyard of terra-cotta roofed apartments, turns out to be a cheerful, clean, well-lighted accommodation, certainly a comfortable refuge in which to relax within this tourist hub. Our hostess is quite gracious and speaks fluent English with a French accent. She lets us know she is available around the clock to assist us during our stay in Florence. We notice the lobby is overflowing with brochures advertising daytrips to the wine country, Tuscan bike tours and trips to Siena, Lucca and other Renaissance and medieval towns. We don't see our hostess again until the afternoon before we depart, when she proclaims: *"We have not seen you two the entire stay!*

You have been on the run, si?!" And later, when we settle the bill the final evening before our early morning departure, she sighs: *"7:00 AM departure?! You poor things!"* It is becoming clear to me that we rise much earlier than many tourists and obviously we don't take advantage of conveniences like taxis and tour packages.

By late afternoon, we're anxious to find Florence's famous Santa Maria del Fiore Cathedral, more commonly known as "The Duomo." We know it is located nearby, for during our trek in from the train station we caught several enticing peeks of the spherical, dome rising high above the cobbled maze. Although it appeared to be in close proximity, our trek this afternoon proves to be yet another labyrinthine challenge within narrow Italian streets. What we thought would take 5 minutes turns into 20. Eventually, we turn a corner into a piazza, and there it appears: the huge cathedral and towering campanile looming larger than life, close within the confines of the relatively small piazza. My heart races and I feel oddly faint as I advance toward the tall marbled structures. I begin to understand how these immense Houses of God might have instilled the "fear of god" in those of god-fearing faith. The exterior walls of the Duomo are extraordinary, boasting intricate tiled patterns using the best quality marbles—Carrara pink, Prato green and Maremma white. Saintly figures reside in ornate niches and within a long frieze that runs across the façade. Round, rose-hued windows must certainly cast a beautiful light within the cathedral's interior. The huge dome itself—or cupola of the cathedral—is the biggest in the world, rising up to the heavens as was the intent of the church. Craning my neck to take it all in, the cathedral and bell tower appear almost out-of-place and overdressed in their awkward juxtaposition to common shops, kiosks and us mere mortals below. We wander up the steps of the cathedral to examine the huge entrance doors with their exquisite brass panels, each carved meticulously in depictions of biblical scenes. As we encircle the sides and back of the Duomo, I see that the marble on the lower half of the exterior is blackened from years of pollution. Scaffolding shows evidence of a major restoration in progress. Tomorrow we plan to climb the 463 steps it takes to get up and back down the cathedral and duomo's interior. But for now a load of dirty laundry awaits, so we grab a quick meal followed by a fabulous first night in Florence surrounded by the spinning machines in a *lavendaria*.

6 Ottobre

Before coming to Italy, Dad and I had both read *Brunelleschi's Dome* by Ross King and had become thoroughly captivated by the story of the building and politics of the enormous dome. In the early 1400's Fillipo Brunelleschi, goldsmith and clockmaker by trade, won the competition to design a 143 foot diameter dome to cover the Santa Maria del Fiore Cathedral. His challenge was to figure out how to create a dome without the use of external supports, such as flying buttresses. In meeting this challenge, Brunelleschi essentially reinvents the field of architecture. Along the way, he invents new tools and equipment necessary to lift massive tons of weight to heights greater than was previously necessary. Brunelleschi constructed the dome using not one but two shells: an outer shell that created a huge exterior sphere and a smaller inner shell that provided partial support as well as being better proportioned to the interior scale of the cathedral. At 9:00 AM this morning, it is this space between the two shells that Dad and I will ascend in our climb to the top of the cathedral's dome.

Arriving early, we begin our ascent by taking a steep, narrow flight of stairs located in the interior and adjacent to the body of the cathedral. By the time we get half-way up the structure, we discover we are able to walk inward toward the cathedral's interior, where we find ourselves on a viewing ledge that encircles the base of the domed interior. Far below us now sit rows of pews and altars and we watch a small mass that is in progress. Directly above us is the interior of Brunelleschi's dome. In essence, we are standing at the very base of the cupola, at eye level of the painted ceiling. We study the elaborate frescoes depicting scenes of heaven and hell. My eyes stay affixed for awhile to a reptilian, horned creature with a devilishly curled tail that is impaling its pitchfork into the neck of some poor mortal. Upbeat biblical scenes such as this can be seen all throughout Italy. I continue my gaze upward: the scenes of death soon replaced by loftier figures of angels and gods until I notice the very peak of the cupola—or *lantern*—where Dad and I will soon emerge. We track back to the narrow flight of stairs and start climbing between the two shells of the duomo: we are now climbing on top of the interior dome, over the painted ceiling and immediately beneath the outer exterior dome. At a landing we pause to catch our breath and peer out one of the dome's portals that offers a great view of Florence. I continue following in Dad's footsteps as the shell arches further upward, the outer dome always just inches above our heads. At last we reach the lantern where we emerge into the brisk morning air onto an outside deck. Florence spreads before us in all directions, a vast sea of terra-cotta tiled rooftops. "Awesome!" is the one word that escapes Dad's lips as he views the city and surrounding Tuscan hillsides. "Maybe this is the best way to see Firenze" I tell him.

Touching down to terra-firma, we head for a cappucino bar, then wander into an outdoor antique market of sorts. Permanent stalls filled with old postcards, lamps, books and bric-a-brac grabs our attention. At a veggie stand advertising *"frutte e verdere"* we point out a bunch of *uva Italia* (large delicious green grapes.) Having by now learned we must *point* or *ask*— but not TOUCH the produce—beneath the watchful eyes of the vender we successfully complete our purchase and press onward. Trekking through the circuitous alleyways of stone, we pass *pasterrias, birrerias, gelatorias, farmacias* and many *porfumerias*, as well as leather shops, high-end clothing stores, jewelry stores and trendy home interior stores. When we reach the streets leading up to the Arno River and the famous Ponte Vecchio Bridge, it's no surprise to see Dad pivot away from the hoardes of *turisti* jumbled around the stalls of jewelry, scarves and curios. I take my cue as we hoof it out of there and find a spot to eat a bite of *pannini*. Seated on a less-traveled arched bridge, we spend our lunch break lulled by the peaceful gliding of rowers in scull boats, the Ponte Vecchio Bridge now a safe and scenic distance.

The Pensione Scoti turns out to be in a great central location. We must have stopped here four times today to regroup, take breaks and drop off or pick up extra layers of clothing. By 5:30 p.m., we add an additional two miles to our long walking day, as we head to the Galleria dell-Accademia, where we waltz right in to see *David*. This is the kind of ease we enjoy when dealing with museums. We are not at all disappointed by *David*. Michelangelo's sculpture is truly a masterpiece, from the exquisitely-defined ribs and relaxed muscles of his marbled torso to the fine pronounced veins of his neck and hands. I think to myself that Michelangelo must have gotten his inspiration from the many beautiful young men of Italia.

The cuisine of Firenze deserves honorable mention. This evening we discover a number of good osteria in the neighborhood on the south side of the Arno. I break my moratorium on eating veal and savor every bite of three tender patties of scaloppini with cooked spinach and soft buffalo mozzarella. Dad orders an al dente linguine with the succulent *Ceps mushrooms*. The hearty Tuscan bread is the best *pane* we will taste during our entire stay in Italy. The vino della regionale in Firenze is Chianti and my ¼ litro for 2.50 E it hits the spot.

This evening I'm reading the Lawrence Block novel that Dad has finished. It is Block's first book, entitled "No Score". Jeez Dad, it's RACEY, I think to myself as I dig into the first chapters. Written almost as a parody—a tongue in cheek commentary during the sexual revolution of the 60's and 70's—it's about a young man who falls into mischief and mayhem, the willing subject of women's amorous desires. It's a fast read and I like the protagonist, Chip Harrison. I notice Dad found a copy of Tim O'Brien's "If I Die in a Combat Zone" in the lobby of Pensione Scoti this afternoon. He tells me he read the book when it was first published in 1969 and was quite moved by it at the time. It's O'Brien's account of a foot soldier serving in the Vietnam War. Dad tells me when the book was released its candid content of the brutal realities of a foot soldier attracted the attention of many anti-war activists and supported all the reasons for the war resistance. I had lived through the Vietnam War era, but didn't read books on the subject until years later. Now, I feel compelled to read O'Brien's book and discuss it with Dad. The vital and youthful energy I feel within the streets of Florence is transporting me back to those days of my youth—the 1970's—a confusing time for me as I was trying to "find myself"—who I was away from the entity of my family. In retrospect, it seemed to be a more carefree time, when I felt lighter and freer. I remember the lottery during the Vietnam War. I had just graduated from high school, when classmates were beginning to receive their numbers and praying to get a high one. The guys I knew did not want to go to Vietnam. None of them wanted to die. I remember a young woman I worked with at Safeway in Santa Cruz. We were both about 19. She was already saving money to buy a house and waiting for her high school sweetheart to return from Vietnam so they could marry. She lived for his letters to arrive in the mail. She was overjoyed—elated—when he finally did return one day, months later, safely in one piece. They were lucky. One of my friends went AWOL. Another developed a debilitating nervous condition from his exposure to Agent Orange. And one acquaintance went totally mad after a tour of duty as a bomber pilot. And in regards to the sexual revolution of the 60's and 70's, well, I had my own free will. When I couldn't convince one of my female friends to move with me to Santa Cruz, it was my boyfriend who gladly raised his hand and volunteered. We didn't get married. That wasn't cool. We found a rental by the beach and adopted a black Labrador puppy. A few years later, Frank received custody of Boo and I moved in with my next love. I had become a serial co-habitator—at least for the time being. As the skies of Firenze begin to darken, I hear "Stairway to Heaven" playing off in the distance. I am 21 again, I'm back in Santa Cruz and the turntable is still circling after a long night of dancing. I fall into slumber lulled by the nostalgic sounds of rock 'n roll.

7 Ottobre

Journal entry reads: *Two more days in Florence. What to do?* Having seen the Duomo and David, we are already seeking escape from the maddening crowds. Dad suggests we pick a town—any town—in the country that is on the train line. Studying the map (a habit that is now bordering on obsessive with him) he suggests a small town called Borgo San Lorenzo ... "an easy hour train-ride away" Dad contends. I'm sure you've all heard of it! Not Siena, or Lucca, or Orvieto or any of those other charming towns of Tuscany advertised in our hotel lobby. No, Borgo San Lorenzo—I read later—is part of the grand prix circuit. My greatest trepidation is that it will just be some unattractive suburb and not a charming village at all.

These feelings quickly subside, however, as our early morning train rolls away from Firenze and winds into the beautiful eastern mountains, in a region called the Mugello. We are transported through vineyards, wineries and mountain villages, as we follow a river and gradually climb in elevation. Arriving to Borgo San Lorenzo, indeed it appears to be an uninteresting suburb, but after walking a mile or more into the *centro antico*, we receive another good ole' dose of old world charm. A stone cathedral, tree-shaded parks and a slower pace draws us in. Locals are dressed casually and nobody seems to speak English, so we keep our mouths shut, short of a quick *giorno!* or *grazie!* An economically robust, small downtown, with not a single unoccupied building, tells us perhaps this is a bedroom community to Florence. Although we have found refuge from the busy streets of Florence, Dad is still dissatisfied: *"On our train ride this morning, we passed a much smaller town called Vicchio"*. He pulls out the map to show me and I realize having missed our opportunity to visit Cuorgne, he still longs to show me a glimpse into small village life. Dad was able to visit Cuorgne in 1969, during an ever-so-brief business trip to Torino and his impressions of family life in the village of his ancestors left a lasting impression. So it is, by mid-day we depart Borgo San Lorenzo and get dropped off in the quaint village of Vicchio nestled in the hillsides. It is early afternoon and most of the stores and restaurants are closed for siesta. Few people are out in the streets and the mood is quite peaceful. A group of four elderly Italian men are seated outside a shop that is closed for mid-day; they play a game of cards at a small table. We linger through the empty streets, pausing at a fenced schoolyard where children play. Dad stoops to return a small toy that two little Italian boys have dropped through a rung in the fence. "Grazie!" they smile at him. "Prego!" he exclaims back, which for some reason makes the boys giggle. We enjoy Vicchio. This is as close as we will get on our trip through Italy to finding small village life. We eat a relaxing meal of pasta at a restaurant not far from the train depot, then return to Florence where the frenzied tourist pace of the afternoon is in full gear.

It is growing dark as we relax this evening in our room. A warm late summer breeze and the aroma of cooking garlic waft through our window, bringing me a sense of well-being. The familiar cacophony of a television program and snatches of conversation tells me a family lives in one of the apartments within our courtyard. From the alleyways, I hear the constant resonance of vespas, people chatting and laughter. The lyrics of a 1970's Jethro Tull tune resounds from speakers somewhere off in the cobbled jungle.

I have trouble sleeping tonight. As I lie here in the same room as my 79 year old dad, I feel distinctly middle-aged. To this very day, 13 years after my surgery, I feel a certain tautness and constriction of my abdomen from the reconstruction that immedi-

ately followed the mastectomy. The plastic surgeon removed a rectus muscle and tissues from my abdomen to create a new left breast, and in doing so gave me a tummy tuck. He slashed a long, wide swath of my abdominal skin and used a piece of it to place a patch over the area once occupied by my left nipple. My torso—like a wetsuit—was pulled together tight and firm. I remember one week prior to the surgery, I had a massage which caused me to deeply relax and take down my guard for the first time since my diagnosis. I broke down emotionally that after- noon and began seriously questioning my decision to have this major reconstructive surgery immediately following the mastec- tomy. How could I allow myself to go through such an invasive and mutilating procedure? Wasn't I going through enough by enduring the mastectomy alone? How vain am I? Maybe not so much vanity as being frightened? Frightened to wake up to one size C-breast adjacent to a flat ribcage without a nipple? I per- sonally didn't want a silicone or saline implant and I resisted a future of dealing with a prosthetic. All the choices seemed lousy to me. I ended up sticking with my original plan to have the sur- gery, however. Although I appreciated the fine work of the sur- geon, as well as the strides that have been made in choices for women faced with breast cancer, the center of my body never felt quite the same after that—nerves had been severed, a muscle removed and my skin had been cinched tightly, leaving me with a core that felt numb and not quite connected anymore.

Several years later, as I trekked with my teammates one long, hot afternoon along the Aconcagua trail, I felt a silence that had replaced our early morning chatter. Following in my teammate's footsteps, I thought of all the missing breasts, the chemo-induced arthritis, the years of hidden scars—our personal maps of our events and histories slashed across our bodies. Although I had *never considered my teammates in such purely physical terms, I was suddenly taken by this macabre imagery as we marched en masse across the barren terrain of the Andes. I felt like the walking wounded—a microcosm of the greater world of humanity itself. It reminded me of a taxi ride that Nancy and I had taken in San Francisco a year earlier. The woman cabbie asked us if we felt women with breast cancer were like the Canaries in the Coal Mines. Explain the metaphor, I pressed her. "Just like the canaries" she began "that were placed in mines to test the levels of toxicity before miners entered, have you ever considered that the millions of women dying with breast cancer are a signal to our society that our species is dying?" This morbid metaphor haunted me for days and has reentered my consciousness from time to time. That afternoon as I hiked alongside my teammates, I began to wonder if we had come to the mountain to reclaim our bodies—to prove to ourselves that we were strong again and more vital than ever. It was more than the personal challenge of the climb, however, that drew us to the expedition: we were climbing to expose the disease to the world. Health care for women had taken a back seat for years; now baby boomers were mobilizing their efforts, asking questions and demanding funding for research, education and support. Some women were exposing their scars—their breasts—their asymmetrical torsos. Breast cancer was no longer a hidden disease where women suffered silently and received little support. Expedition Inspiration had set a goal of 2.3 million dollars—$100 per foot of the mountain. It was a dynamic way to feel a vital part of making a difference.*

I learned much from my teammates and their personal challenges. Many had not opted for reconstructive surgery. Some had fared well with their partners, while others endured difficult separations and divorce, their husbands repulsed by the loss of

a breast. How great it felt then to come together on the moun-
tain, suspending from our cares, trekking upward, each of us in
excellent fitness and lofty spirits, simply enjoying being alive,
well and in the great outdoors.

8 Ottobre

Since Dad has got the train system pretty well wired, we decide
to flee town again and catch a 9:00 AM—this time to explore
the medieval hilltop village of Siena. For over an hour, we ride
the rail, as hillsides of scenic Tuscan countryside and terraced
vineyards roll by our windows. When we reach Siena, we disembark at a train and bus station located several miles below the
city. Siena is perched high above on three steep ridges and our
greatest challenge of the day is catching the correct bus up to the
medieval town. Since neither of us understands the ticket clerk's
directions, we simply board the first bus that arrives. The bus
goes up hill alright, but then bypasses the *centro antico* altogether, taking a wide sweep through the hillsides past a hospital
complex, a number of student apartments and several universi-
ties. Somehow, Dad determines where to disembark and catch
the right bus back to the *center antico*. I have no idea how he
figured it out.

Siena turns out be an extraordinarily scenic and interesting
hill town, completely intact as it was in the 12th and 13th centuries. Red brick and terra-cotta roof-tiled dwellings blanket the
three ridge tops and cobbled alleyways serpentine through the
uneven, hilly terrain. We duck through small, brick passage-
ways and crest up and over alleyways, past tiny homes, restaurants and by a few hubs of stores geared toward tourism. At any
number of junctures we find ourselves with some dramatic
view, be it the magnificent cathedral and campanile that rise

ominously from another ridge, or a spectacular view of the Tuscan countryside below, as seen from within the brick wall that surrounds the hilltop city. I imagine what it might be like to stay at a three, four or five star hotel (I imagine this a lot!) We trek over to the next ridge where we join other *turisti* to gape at Siena's cathedral and *campanile*. It seems futile to snap a photograph, since I could not possibly fit the towering structures within the frame of my lens. We spend time perusing impressive art of the Renaissance period in one of the many museums. While I'm staring at about the 50th life-size picture of J.C. nailed to the cross, Dad appears next to the portrait, flails his skinny arms out in the symbol of the cross and smiles at me with a devious grin, his eyes peaking out from beneath his green beanie. I feel like I'm touring Italy with Father Guido Sarducci, as it is now my turn to dart away and ditch Dad.

By mid-day, tourists congregate at *Piazzo del Campo,* the town's huge central square. I feel as if I am standing in an immense, shallow bowl of mortared bricks that have been pressed into the lopsided hilltop basin. Siena is where I begin noticing statues of *La Lupa*, the she-wolf and nursemaid, who is suckled by the twins, Romulus and Remes. Roman legend has it that Romulus is the founder of Rome, while Remes plays a much lesser role, having been killed by his twin. Some versions of the tale refer to *La Lupa* as the mother of Rome. I wonder how many rich, historical details we float by in our intrepid wanderings. I would love at least one more day in Siena, but all too soon, it is almost time to take off again.

The weather in this hilltop town is too cool to dine *al fresco* and neither of us is interested in eating at the outdoor tables set around the periphery of the piazza where groups of *turisti* congregate. Instead, we duck into an *osteria* that is not set up for the popular al fresco dining experience. The brick-walled interior is rather dark, but cozy, with not a soul in sight except the young lady who waits on us. The chef turns out to be our waitress's mother, who whips up a lovely, fluffy asparagus soufflé and a polenta with grilled vegetables. Dad successfully navigates our way back to the bus stop where we wait to catch a ride down the hill to the train depot. Flyers stapled on a kiosk at the bus stop advertising classes in Tai Chi, Martial Arts, Massage, Art and Italian Language classes are evidence that we are in a liberal and language arts college town.

It's 5:00 pm by the time we board our commuter train back to *Firenze*. Our short trip through the Tuscan Region and Renaissance world is quickly winding down. I realize there is so much art and sights I had originally intended to visit while in *Firenze*; finding it all within the intense tourist hub turned out to be another story. Tomorrow we will head 500 miles south to Naples, closer to the boot of the country. My traveling friends have warned me: *Naples? You are staying in Naples? It's an armpit! Stay in Sorrento. Don't stay in Naples. Watch your pack. Be careful. It's a dump.*

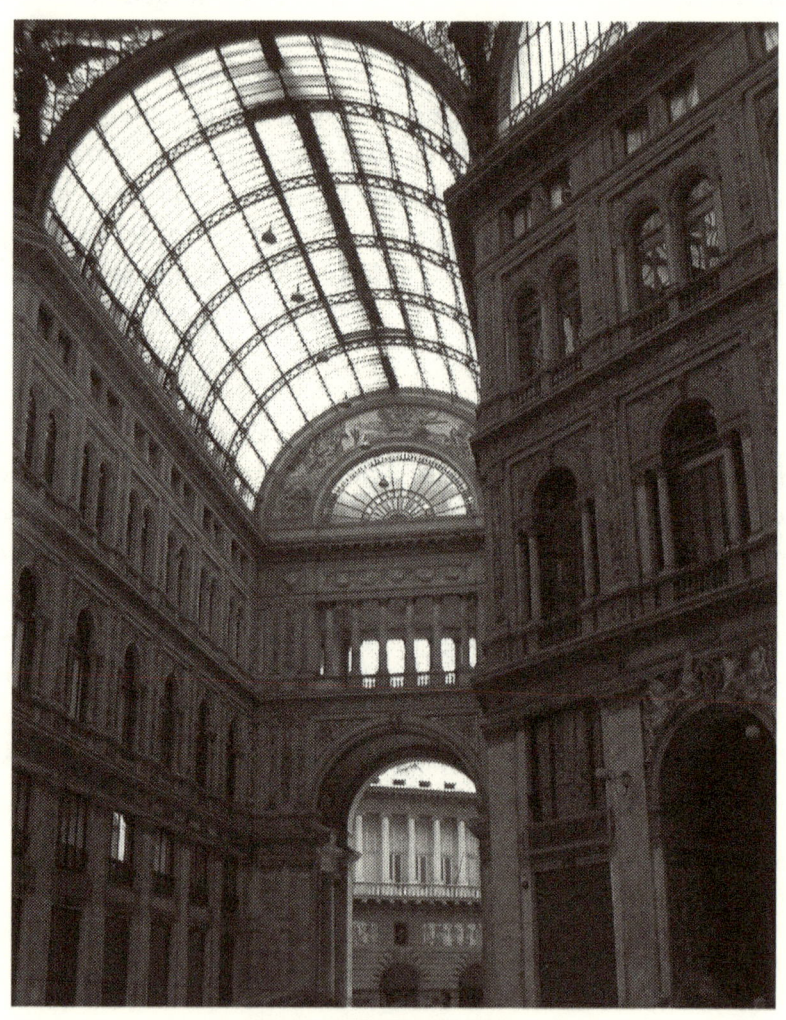

Napoli—Ceiling of Galleria

Napoli

9 Ottobre

This morning we board The Eurostar (the ES) which will transport us 490 miles south to Naples. The ES is a sleek, fast moving train with immense, clean windows, a great way to take in the countryside. Our route today will take us along the spine of the country, through Central and Southern Italy, following the west side of the Appenines Mountain Range. The ES glides—practically flies—at 100mph. When we reach the suburbs of Rome, we notice that other than a few shabby-looking trailer parks and shacks, we have seen no obvious signs of poverty during these two weeks of travel. Italy, so far, appears to be economically stable, and the north especially affluent. Where are all the teams of con-artists and beggars we have read about? Perhaps we will see them in Naples or later in downtown Rome. As we continue due south the terrain grows drier, rockier and barren. I'm surprised at the number of marble quarries we pass. Evidence of substantial harvesting can be seen in the railroad yards—thick, long slabs of white marble are stacked in piles ready for shipping.

I know about rock quarries. At least that's what I felt I was facing that first day on Mt. Aconcagua. On Day One, the Trek Team took turns being shuttled in the back of an old pickup truck to a spot at 8,000 feet where we would begin our three-day trek to Base Camp. It was summer in Argentina; the skies were clear and the weather already warming. Standing within the dusty, rock-laden bowels of the Andes, all we could see before us were huge mountains of talus and scree. I understood now the references made to the mountain: "the giant slag heap" and "the Stone Sentinel." The women and mountain guides of the Trek Team joined hands and formed a circle for five minutes of silence before beginning the long-awaited journey. We thought of our summit team, who had reached Base Camp by this time. Enthusiastic chatter filled the air as we took off single file behind our leader, Mark "Tuck" Tucker. Elated to finally take our first steps toward the mountain, I followed in Sue Ann's footsteps, as I listened to the tinkling of a small bell she had laced to her right boot and noticed a tiny Earth Flag embroidered on her pack.

Our trek into Base Camp, located at 14,000 feet, would take three days to reach, with an elevation gain of 6,000 feet. "Base Camp" is where climbing expeditions set up camp to rest and to function as a lower-based-station—a home-base of sorts to the upper camps. From Base, the climb toward the summit becomes increasingly difficult and climbers no longer utilize mules to carry their supplies. Instead, they use the strength of their own backs to pack gear up to the higher camps. The common practice for climbing above Base Camp is referred to as "climbing high and sleeping low." This approach toward reaching the summit allows for optimal acclimatization and the easier managing of gear as you move camp upward. At Base Camp, for example, our summit team would pack tents and essential gear, climb to Camp I located at 16,250 feet, then descend back to Base Camp to sleep that night. The following day, encumbered with less weight, they would ascend once again to Camp I, where they would then sleep. They repeat this routine as they make their next ascent from Camp I to Camp II, located at 19,000 feet. Then, finally, once a decent "window of weather" presents itself, the summit attempt is made in one, long grueling day beginning well before the crack of dawn, in order to reach 23,000 feet and return to 19,000 before dusk. Brutal.

The Trek Team's three-day climb to Base Camp proved to be one long, arduous march over boulder-laden, dusty paths, broken up by occasional and exciting stream crossings. Our daily routine on the mountain rarely faltered: Each morning we broke camp, packed our duffels and ate a quick breakfast. By 7:00 AM, our fearless leader, Tuck, gathered us together to review the territory ahead. While Tuck advised, the team sucked down water, strapped on our packs and slathered sunscreen on our exposed skin. We each carried about 15 to 20 pounds on our backs. The rest of our gear was carried by mules that were herded by a few Argentine gauchos. The muleteer didn't actually hike with us; in fact, we only crossed paths with them maybe once or twice during the day. When we spotted the gauchos and the dustbowl of kicking mules rounding a bend, quickly we jumped off the trail to let the stampede gallop by. It was clear who had the right of way on the mountain. We usually beat the muleteer to our campsite each evening. Filthy, sweaty and exhausted from ten hours on the trail, we would rest against our packs waiting for the gauchos to arrive so we could collect our big, canvas duffels, set up our tents and change out of our dirty clothing. When the muleteer finally did get to camp, it was total pandemonium as a number of the feisty beasts tried escaping up the mountainsides, kicking wildly at the burdens on their backs. The gauchos rounded them up in a whirling dustbowl as we held back, waiting for our gear. It wasn't until the gauchos tied a down jacket or serape around the mule's head that the beasts began to settle down. Once the beasts calmed down, the gauchos unleashed the 60 lb. duffels from their backs, dropping them recklessly to the ground below, where my teammates and I could finally dash over to retrieve them. Some of us felt sorry for the mules, but were relieved to have their assistance during our ascent up the "sentinel of stone."

Each day as we ascended higher, the panorama of the Andes became more spectacular. Vistas of undulating mountains and craggy cliffs unfolded as far as the eye could see, in an earthy palate of gold, ambers and burnt sienna. Occasional drippings of patina gleamed against the mountainsides, while the entire range contrasted magnificently against a vast, Cerulean blue sky. It wasn't until the end of the second day of our trek, while rounding a final bend into camp that Mt. Aconcagua came looming into our sight. I remember distinctly how she appeared before us, as if she had been awaiting our arrival for many years. Magnificent, snow-covered sentinel of stone, she was far grander in scale than anything I had ever seen. The entire Trek Team halted to gape at her imposing stature. By now I had learned to respect nature. Nature was in charge. I had been tossed off kayaks in a wild river and churned up and down within the violent undertow of the Pacific. As a child, a cloud burst open on me during a walk home from school, drenching me like a drowned rat. I knew nature could turn on me at any moment. And now, here she loomed, inviting us to scale her body, daring us to come closer. We could see that her peak was obscured in a menacing flurry of clouds and we knew the Summit Team was up there somewhere. Tuck made radio contact with the Summit Team a couple hours later. Peter informed him that they had reached Camp I at 16,250 feet and were hunkered down in their tents waiting out a snow storm. Laura got on the airwaves and screamed: "Hey team! It's as cold as Siberia up here. We're all ok, though—no problems, so far." Relieved to hear familiar voices, it was good to finally make contact with our teammates. It would be a number of days yet before we were physically reunited and our Summit Team had yet to face the ascent to 19,000 feet and the final hump up to the top.

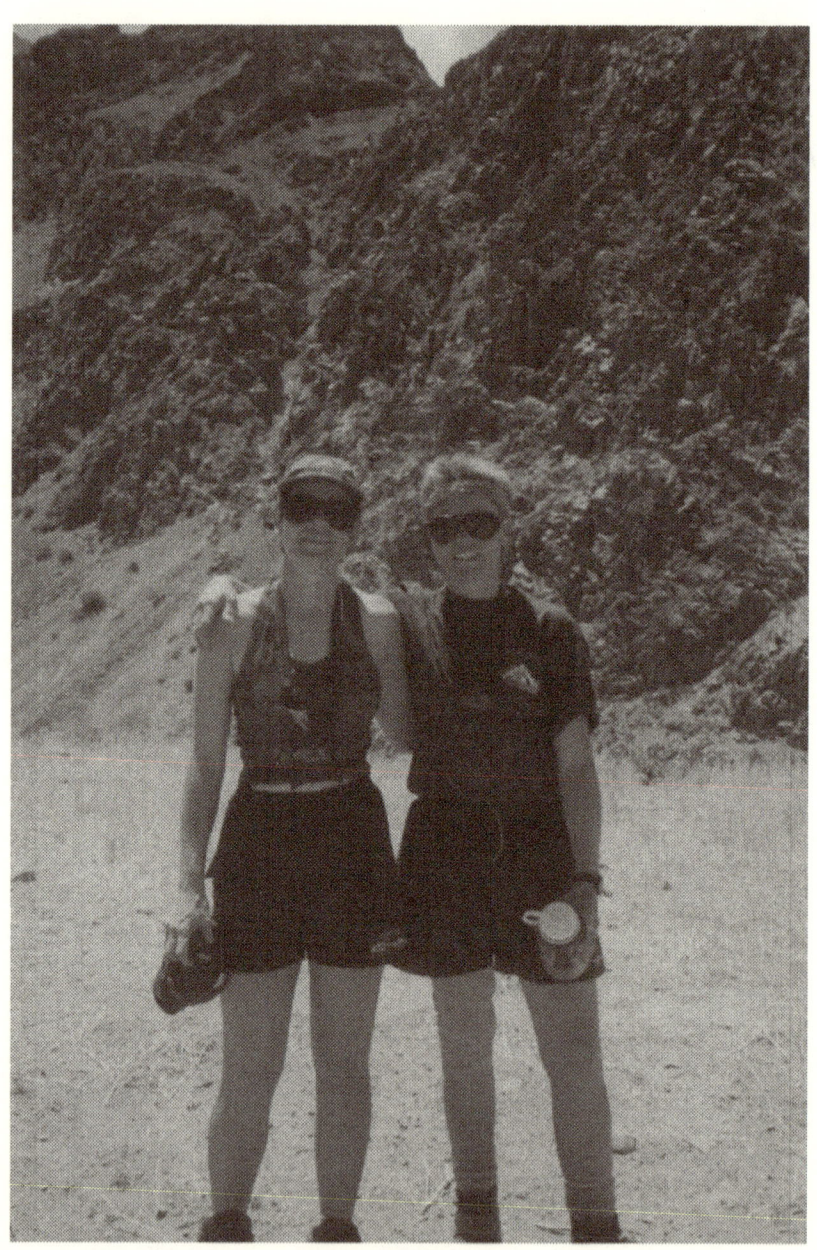

Nancy and me

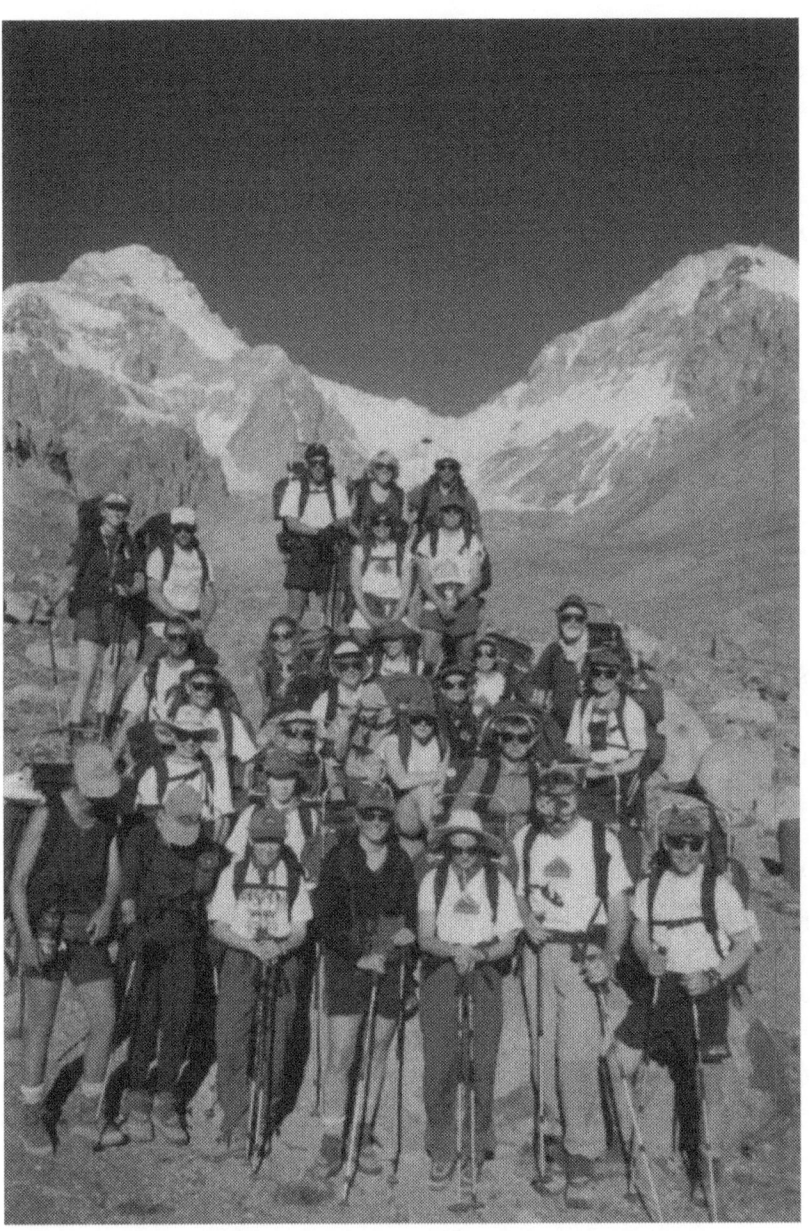

Expedition Inspiration Team

Dad nudges me awake. "We're getting close to Naples," he's studying the map of the downtown area. He reminds me that Naples—or Napoli—is the third largest city in Italy, with a population of 2 million in the general area. One-third of the people are unemployed "That's about 9% higher than during the Great American Depression" Dad helps me put the poverty of the area into perspective. Travel literature promotes Napoli for its beautiful natural setting located in the Gulf of Naples. Mt. Vesuvius rests in close proximity, as do the islands of Capri and Ischia. I read that we can easily board the Circumvesuviana Railway that follows the bay from Napoli to Pompeii then continues around the bay to the charming cliff town of Sorrento. Words describing the character of Napoli include: chaotic traffic, colorful street life, sunny climate, friendly people, great cuisine and armpit.

It was Dad's idea to come to Napoli; I, on the other hand, had some trepidation. Most people I talked to go to Napoli to take a boat or train to somewhere else. We, however, are going to stay for three nights. I eventually became more intrigued with the south, when I read Thomas Harris' *Pompeii*, a historical fiction that takes place four days leading up to the fatal eruption of Vesuvius in 79 AD. My curiosity of Napoli became further piqued by descriptions of the colorful Spaccanapoli District in which our pensione is located: *full of lengthy, narrow alleys and a lively street life* the guide book promises. At the very least our hotel room is a mere 65 Euro a night and we will be within easy traveling distance of Pompeii and the islands. I begin to shrug off people's accounts of street crime, con artists and terms like "dump" and decide they were probably simply accustomed to higher class travel. Besides, how bad can it be?

As our train enters greater Napoli, we roll by blocks upon blocks of tall, boxy, non-descript apartment projects that are packed together like one, huge, ugly erector-set in the streets and hills above the port area. Everywhere we look hang lines of laundry—the unofficial flag of Napoli—draped across cracked, gray exterior walls. When we disembark from the Eurostar at the Napoli train station, with packs on back and neck purse tucked securely beneath my shirt, I stand hyper-alert and ready to take the city on. Nothing, however, prepares me for what lies ahead. On this Saturday afternoon, the moment we step foot outside the train station, the scene is full-tilt boogie. Taxis are lined five lanes deep outside the station, ready to snare *turisti*. We're barely out on the streets before we notice beggars and homeless people. Cars, taxis and buses vie for position against a cacophony of honking horns. For the first time on this trip I am intently watching Dad's back, as we hightail it down a sidewalk that follows the Corso Umberto I, an incredibly wide, heavily trafficked thoroughfare. My whole body tenses up and my determined stride warns the masses "don't mess with me!" as we begin to shoulder through blocks of aggressive, barking street merchants. The vehicle traffic seems chaotic and disorganized and the boulevard we follow is about six lanes deep and a challenge to run across, especially since traffic lights are scarce. We don't see many bicycles here—mostly cars, motorcycles, taxis and a good deal of patrolling *polizia*. We both remain hyper-alert in the coming days, especially when we navigate the Corso Umberto I that runs near the port and train station area.

Once we're safely across the boulevard, we enter a grid of lengthy alleyways that move upward toward the Spaccanapoli District. The melee of humanity decreases by a few decibels and before long we find ourselves within the boxy neighborhoods we noticed on the train ride in. I am taken aback by the trash-laden streets and the sight of a few overflowing dumpsters. The streets of Firenze seem benign in comparison. Our pensione is located on a long, cobbled alleyway darkened by tall apartment projects. The street is filled with clusters of small shops and stalls, selling pizza by the slice, pastries, books and inexpensive scarves and clothing. Our first reaction when we reach the Albergo Duomo is one of foreboding. Housed in one of the many tall buildings, we gaze at the 15 foot high steel gates butted up to the sidewalk. Pressing a buzzer, located beneath the watchful eye of a security camera, the steel gate creaks open to a gloomy courtyard occupied by three big, black motorcycles—real hogs compared to the small vespas that filled the sidewalks and streets of Milano and Firenze. Climbing three flights of concrete stairs, we are greeted by a friendly, handsome Italian man, one of three brothers who own the establishment. We are delighted at the cleanliness and tidiness we discover within. Our room is spacious, yet somewhat dark due to the narrow alleyway and tall apartments that are practically an arm's-length out our window.

We have the afternoon ahead of us, so I suggest we explore part of the city by making the Museo Archeological Nazionale our first sojourn. I entice Dad to go, by reading to him about the many pre-Christian Greek and Roman antiquities at the museum, as well as it housing much of what was unearthed from the city of Pompeii. Trekking down the alleyway outside our pensione, past food stalls and chatting locals, Napoli reminds me of one, big outdoor party. I feel oddly relaxed amidst the teeming humanity and casbah-like atmosphere. The locals seem really down to earth—a number of them so much so they lie prostrate on the sidewalks and in parks—and it's barely 2:00 PM. We reach the avenue leading up to the Museo

Archeologica, where I notice care has been taken in cleaning up the trash in the immediate vicinity of the museum. The Museo Archeologica turns out to be the best museum we will visit on our entire stay in Italy. Only a handful of visitors are here this afternoon. It feels like a quiet and moving sanctuary within the tumult of the surrounding city streets. The afternoon sunlight streams in from a spacious courtyard that illuminates marble statues of Isis, Aphrodite and Athena. We're both elated to see something other than J.C., Madonna and Bambino and scenes of heaven and hell. A phenomenal creation fills the entire corner of one room: the Toro Franese (Farnese Bull) from 3rd Century AD. Chiseled from one single, huge block of magnificently textured marble, the piece depicts the death of Dirce, Queen of Thebes. The wild bull, to which the queen is tied, is dramatically central to the carving. His forelegs kick in midair, while the five other characters of the myth surround the beast in an exquisitely intertwined scene of marble. We wander over to the rooms that house the artifacts unearthed from Pompeii and Herculaneum—the two cities destroyed by Vesuvius in 79 AD. The collection includes large mosaic scenes entirely created by miniscule, colorful tiles, as well as paintings and frescos that were removed from the walls and floors of Pompeii's homes and temples. We visit the *Gabinetto Segreto* (the Secret Room) which displays the ancient porn from Pompeii's brothels and private homes. Menus for brothel clients depict erotic positions. Souvenirs for patrons of the brothels, sculpted in the shapes of phallic symbols, leave no question as to the character of the destroyed city.

Emerging from the quiet museum, out into the busy streets of Napoli, I am taken aback by the numbers of overweight Italians we pass this afternoon. It's nothing like some of the obesity I have observed in the U.S., but there is still a distinct general difference in girth between the people of the south and north of Italy. I notice that the delis and stores of Napoli are a far cry from those of Torino and Florence. The succulent hens and artichoke tortes of the North have been replaced by fried foods, particularly French fries and greasy take-out pizza. We notice the American term "Fast Food" plastered on signs throughout Napoli. The pastries displayed in bakery windows look sugary and airy. Despite the abundance of fatty fast food, we have heard about great sit-down cuisine, and that the pizza—which originated in Napoli—can be quite good. We enter an appealing restaurant, packed with a lively clientele and order the original traditional version of pizza called The Margharita. The Margharita has a simple topping of buffalo mozzarella, olive oil and fresh tomatoes and basil. The pizza is excellent, especially the crust, which has a chewy, puffy consistency reminding me of a cross between East Indian bread and a Mexican flour tortilla.

The streets are swamped with locals. Not only do they hang out on the sidewalks, they linger about the streets chatting, gesticulating and carrying on. As we navigate our way back toward the Spaccanopoli neighborhood, suddenly a motorcade of polizia, sirens screaming, come roaring around a bend in the street, quickly separating the crowds back to the sidewalks like the parting of the Red Sea. I had read somewhere that the current mayor of Napoli is on a serious campaign to clean up the crime in the city and that as a result the street scene had been improving. I'm assuming this macho assertion of authority we just witnessed is meant to serve as a pre-Saturday night warning.

Unlike the reserved presence of the crowds in the North, Napoli is boisterous, like an open air carnival. The mere masses

of people who roam the streets add to the chaos. Seating ourselves on a bench at a spacious piazza, we take a gelato break,
and spend time watching a young man and his young son kicking
around a soccer ball. A teen-aged couple wanders over and put
on an impressive display of drama as they exchange accusations,
tongues wagging and fingers pointing at each other. They are lit-
erally in each other's faces, then within minutes all is well with
one big, mushy kiss and embrace. Dad laughs and tells me they
are putting on a show for us and then I remember what I had read
about the "natural theatricality of the locals in Napoli." I remain
overwhelmed by the shear volume of people moving about me
and am repulsed by the trash that seems to be strewn everywhere. Dad appears unaffected and calm by this environment as
he continues to enjoy watching the boy and his father who kick
the soccer ball around the piazza. "Notice that woman?!" Dad
nods toward a tiny, elderly lady who promenades through the
crowds. Wearing a modest dress, jacket, and low heels, she steps
right over a pile of litter and continues to proudly forge ahead,
body upright and her spirit true to the passagietta.

With dusk upon us, we are anxious to get back to our pensione. There's no way to return, however, without taking the
lengthy, dark alleyway that seems to go on for about a mile. We
pass street venders and groups of locals chatting, drinking and
partying, as they gear up for Saturday night. Cooking on outdoor stoves fills a few pockets of the neighborhood with smoke.
Motorcycles frequently roar down the alley: we jump out of the
way as one zooms by us. There are no street lamps in sight and
with dark now upon us—be it ever so unfashionable—I wish I
was sporting my florescent biking vest.

Safely back in our room at 7:30 PM, the street noise of the night seems to go on for hours. These high rises are packed so closely together, I feel merely an arm's distance from my neighbors. Through our open window blasts the cacophony of a blaring television program, family conversations, children still at play and the roar of motorcycles that zoom through the narrow alleyway. Later, a man breaks out into song and then I hear someone coughing up phlegm so clearly it's as if he's sharing our room. When I mention to Dad that I'm wondering how I will ever get any sleep this evening, he responds that for the first time on our trip he takes comfort in the sounds generated by families instead of tourists. He falls asleep rocked by the vital sounds of the city, as I lie awake for several hours, pondering how we will spend the next two days in Napoli.

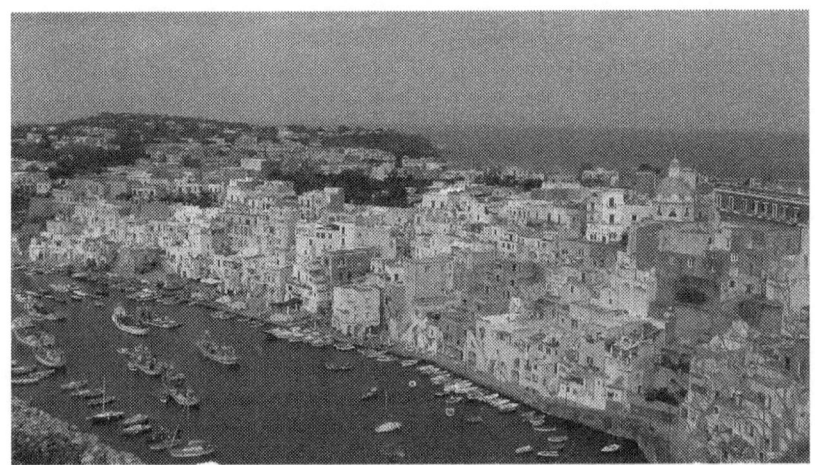

Procida

10 Ottobre

An easy agreement has been reached that the best way to spend the remaining two days in Napoli is to get out of town as early as possible and arrive back to our room just before dark. At 7:30 this morning we head for the port where we plan to take a hydrofoil across the bay to the island of Procida. Kicking our way through litter, and stepping over piles of feces, we notice that the few dumpsters available to the citizens are now spilling over with trash. Discarded crushed beer cans, Styrofoam cups, empty cigarette packs and chewed cobs of corn (some of the healthier vender fare) all add to the city's ambience. It's really disgusting. By the looks of the streets, it appears that everyone had a good Saturday night. Dad philosophically muses that this is nothing compared to the city of Manama, Bahrain where Mom and he lived for almost two years in the late 1970's.Unlike Napoli, which appears to have some garbage pickup, Bahrain had no services whatsoever, at least none that Dad can recall. He recounts the trails of trash in the streets and passing the carcass of a dead goat each morning as he took his daily jog. The carcass decayed quickly over time in the hot desert environment, so why bother moving it, Dad contends. Each time I step over a new pile of shit and wince, Dad continues to wax philosophic: *"You're here to suck up the culture, Claudia. Suck it up!"*

We find a cappuccino bar on our way to the port. It's clean and tidy and run by friendly Neapolitans. We've noticed once we step inside off the littered streets, that the cafes, hotels, and shops are spotless. Dad recounts this same phenomenon in Manama: the homes, shops and businesses were quite clean, but the moment you stepped foot on the street, rats would cross your path and trails of litter abounded. *You just get used to it*, Dad reminisces. He got used to it. Mom got used to it. You just go on living. What can you do when there is no city infrastructure to handle the trash? I don't know how often garbage is collected in Naples but obviously it's a big problem. I read later that there is nowhere to ship the trash and there is a lack of space in Naples for reprocessing centers. Regional officials for years have been trying to build two large incinerators, but their efforts have been blocked by residents who don't want the plants in their neighborhoods and environmentalists who don't want the plants at all. Schools and open-air markets have been shut down at times as health measures. Blockades have been erected by angry residents to keep municipal authorities from reconverting local warehouses to temporary trash depots. The Mafia has been blamed. There seem to be no easy answers to the refuse problem of a couple million people who are packed in such close proximity.

When we reach the Porto di Napoli I notice it is fairly free of litter. "They keep the tourist areas clean" Dad explains to me. A grand fortress—Castel Nuovo—is perched at the edge of the port. It looks odd resting there next to the gargantuan cruise ships, hydrofoils and ferries that dock to unload tourists and commuters. We watch a cruise line of tourists streaming off one of the ships and scatter into the streets of Napoli. I wonder where their captain sends them for their daily outing. There must be an attractive route through town somewhere—perhaps to the castle, then over to the adjoining palace and onward to the Galleria Umberto ... yes that must be the route. Or do they venture to the Museo Archeological and perhaps stop at a pizza stand. I can only imagine the tourists' alarm at navigating the heavily trafficked streets, not to mention the shock of wading through the litter and turd-filled sidewalks. And won't some of them easily get lost and disoriented within the impossible web of alleyways? Later in the day, indeed, one extremely distressed tourist asks us for directions to the dock where she is slated to return within the next ten minutes. Neither Dad nor I are in anyway envious of these cruise goers as we watch them scurry in all directions away from the port.

Gliding across the bay toward the island this morning, the views from the hydrofoil are spectacular. The Gulf of Napoli is dominated by sheer cliffs that look dark purple from a distance and Mt. Vesuvius reigns central to the coastline. We arrive an hour later to the island of Procida. Modest, sea-worn stucco homes, shops and cafes blanket the cliff sides and line the quaint working harbor. Small fishing boats and heaps of netting fill the shorelines. We take our time ascending alleyways that wind upward through cliffy neighborhoods of stucco homes. In this warm, balmy, southern climate we notice hibiscus, bougainvillea, wild morning glories, succulents, grapefruit trees and cheerful red hot pepper plants. Eventually, we crest upon a ridge, and saunter out to headlands where an old weathered fortress faces the sea. The winds are brisk up on the precipice and we decide to head back down toward a small harbor below, where we can spot market umbrellas being erected outside a few cafes. Trekking steeply down more streets jumbled with white stucco homes, we reach the harbor and seat ourselves at a table *al fresco.* While waiting for our *due cappucini,* I notice the cats on this island look scrawny and unhealthy. They shield themselves from the winds by lying beneath the hulls of small boats on the beach and within nooks and crannies of homes and shops. Yesterday, I learned that Procida is where the movie *Il Postino* was filmed. I thoroughly enjoyed this movie about a postman who delivers mail to the famous poet—and communist—Pablo Naruda, who was granted political exile on a small island village of Italy. The mild-mannered postman is a big fan of Naruda's—whose romantic prose is popular with the women of the day. The postman's sole desire is to emulate Naruda's style in order to capture the heart of Beatrice, the fetching young waitress who works and lives at the village bar. I had recommended this film to Dad prior to our trip to Italy, and he too enjoyed it, taking on some of the postman's understated dialect such as "giorno!" instead of "buon giorno." Sipping our cappucino, I notice the long, narrow stretch of beach before us looks similar to the one on which the post-man, Beatrice, as well as Naruda, all strolled at some point during the film. Turning around to the sign above our café it reads: *"La Locanda del Postino."* As kismet would have it, we are seated at the movie setting of the village and bar. We spend the remainder of our day lingering the hillside neighborhoods and taking in the ocean views and sea breezes. Back at the portside of the island we seek out lunch, intentionally avoiding the more crowded restaurants, even though the meals we spot look mighty appetizing. Instead, we share a long lunch right next to a table of *guardia coasteria (*the Italian coast guard.) Of course, Dad loves it. The jovial atmosphere of the restaurant is made warmer by a meal of fresh calamari and spaghetti alla carbonera e *due insalati misti e due birre.*

A late afternoon return on the hydrofoil dumps us back in the streets of Napoli by 6:00 PM. The port area is as lively as ever and the vehicle traffic is hectic and noisy. This time we attempt a less-direct route to our hotel, along the Castel Nouva and uphill toward the grand Galleria. I notice the streets are kept in pristine condition on this particular stretch through the city. When we reach the Galleria, some locals are setting up for a fashion show. A group of teenaged girls queue up to promenade a cat walk that is located in the central rotunda. An enthusiastic audience is seated and standing around the stage, while music is blasting from a couple of loud speakers. Fashion in Napoli seems to be a whole different ballgame from the North. I've been noticing window displays are full of nothing but cheaply made, slinky, risqué women's clothing. The girls in this evening's show simply wear blue jeans and slinky blouses. They seem to be enjoying themselves. We exit the Galleria back into the great cobbled outdoors and eventually come upon a spacious piazza. Smack dab in the center of the square a small scruffy boy sits cross-legged on a warn blanket, cradling a tiny, wire-haired mutt in his lap. The boy's father cranks the volume of a boom box that emits the tinny sound of rock and roll as he encourages his son to SMILE and perform for the passersby. The child plants a permanent grin on his face and frenetically begins orchestrating the wiry paws of his dog to the rhythm of the scratchy music. An aluminum can for tips sits at his feet and a single shopping cart of their belongings rests nearby. I am sad-dened as I consider the boy's existence. At least it is warm in the south. People can sleep outdoors. I've read that the street scene during the night in Napoli can get pretty edgy, but we're not sticking around to find out. We locate a store near our neighborhood, buy some snacks, navigate through gangs of young adults clustered along the alleyways, hit the street buzzer outside of our hotel, wait for the steel gate to slowly creak open, scale the three flights of stairs, quickly smile *Buona Sera* to the Italian guy in our lobby, take two hallways back to our room, tightly deadbolt the door behind us and hunker down for another early evening, prisoners in our own abode.

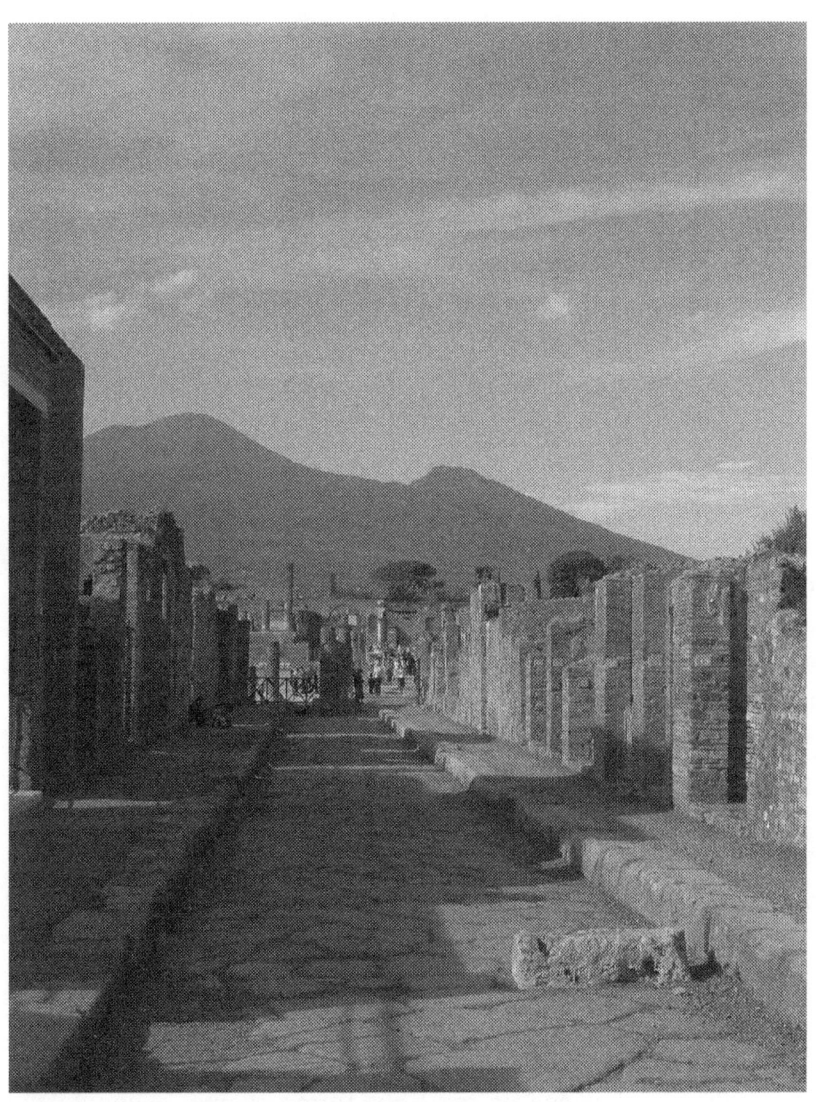

Pompeii

11 Ottobre

The sky is filled with billowing clouds so we purchase two cheap umbrellas at the port, and then buy a mediocre cappuccino with a disgustingly sweet pastry. Although I would truly like to see Pompeii on our final day in the Gulf of Napoli, considering the threat of rain we have settled on Sorrento instead. I'm surprised Dad is willing to go to this tourist town. Perhaps part of the appeal is another ride across the bay on the hydrofoil. In regards to our decision to visit Sorrento, Dad assures me, "… besides, Pompeii is probably nothing more than a bunch of big holes in the ground."

As the hydrofoil hauls us out of the port, from our view off the back deck, Napoli begins to recede. Before she disappears altogether, I notice sprawling greenbelts surrounding the greater downtown area and what look like mansions with manicured lawns near dramatic cliffs overlooking the bay. It appears to be a city where a lot of money is collected in the hands of a few. After an early morning rain—and a good distance from the messy streets of Napoli—everything sparkles. Our boat flies by Mt. Vesuvius and follows the beautiful Sorrentine Peninsula where colorful homes are perched atop sheer cliffs that rise straight up from the sea. Dad is delighted to be standing on the outside deck, within the elements. He balances himself with legs planted firmly in a wide stance, arms clasped behind his back as we speed across the gulf. "This is how we stood in the Navy" he informs me as his light frame seems to handle the wind with ease. Nervously, I duck into the protected area of the hydrofoil and attempt to encourage Dad back inside, but he doesn't budge until the boat nears Sorrento.

When we reach the harbor nestled well below the cliff top village, we disembark and take in the sea breezes at an outdoor café. Just two minutes into our *due cappucini*, sheets of rain begin pounding down. Tourists at the harbor scatter like cockroaches and a couple of waiters immediately roll back the overhead canopy under which we sit. Shop owners frantically move their wares inside as Dad and I dash for the shelter of a nearby tourist store. The female proprietor—anxious to shut the overhead sliding door—gestures us to hurry inside and then battens down the hatches while the rain keeps hammering down.

Smart move to shut a woman in a store, I think, as I begin eyeing the aisles of merchandise. Within ten minutes I buy an inexpensive yellow rain jacket and take this rare opportunity of being around clothing to purchase an Italian scarf. As quickly as the showers began, they pass, and we are out in the streets again where we join a busload packed with tourists heading uphill to Sorrento. Several cramped minutes later, we step off the bus into the streets of a community that screams WEALTH. Sprawling, manicured lawns and meticulously painted stucco exteriors grace the hillsides. City blocks are lined with upscale shops and are overflowing with a melee of *turisti*. "We may as well be in Carmel! "Dad complains immediately in reference to the affluent, seaside artist's community of California. So, as usual, we skip any form of shopping and instead we mosey over to a small park to stare at some pigeons gathered at a fountain. Standing idly in rain-soaked grass, I begin to tell Dad about a dream I had last night. In my dream I was writing a book. I remember feeling grungy, tired, out-of-sorts—perhaps due to the culmination of days spent hiking cobbled streets and nights sleeping upon narrow beds. Mom was in my dream and she was pressing me for the title of my book. Hoping it would be clever, I quickly responded "Rocks in my Pockets!" to which she seemed pleased. I could feel small pebbles in my toes and in one of my pockets was a cache of rocks. "Uh huh" Dad responds absentmindedly as he continues to stare at the pigeons. Then he asks me, "Do you think the birds are any better off NOT KNOWING about Pompeii?" Something tells me a visit to the old ruins is not on Dad's agenda today. "Well, maybe they ARE better off" I indulge Dad in his musings. Perhaps all the facts and information we accumulate simply weigh us down, rendering us flightless. Then I consider how unencumbered I have felt these past weeks, with nothing more than 12 lbs. to carry, a good traveling companion and a healthy sense of adventure and humor.

By now the skies have cleared and it turns into one of those salubrious days that follow a good, cleansing rain, so we decide to attempt an excursion to Pompeii, after all. Trekking back through a stream of tourists and hoofing it down several city blocks, we locate the Circumvesuvian Train Depot in time to catch a mid-day departure. Within the hour, we are chugging along the Gulf of Napoli on a truly spectacular stretch of sheer cliffs. The train winds high above the bay, through dense vegetation, broken up by quaint villages. We sit across from a middle-aged American couple who have been staying in Sorrento for two nights. When I ask how they like Sorrento, the woman quickly responds how enjoyable the quiet of their hotel has been, following two hectic nights in Rome. She explains the stress of having navigated Rome's congested airport, dealing with the packed subway system and waiting in long museum lines. She goes on about how her husband and she had not visited Rome since 1974 and are now disappointed by the number of pizza stands that have sprung up since. *"Thirty years ago we came across only one!"* she lamented. *"I asked a pizzeria manager if the increase of stands was in response to American tourists and he insisted no, that the pizza originated in Naples and had simply taken it's time to spread to Rome. "* She wasn't buying his theory, however, and suspects the burgeoning pizzeria business is a response to globalization and American tourism. I begin to wonder if this couple is trying to relive a trip to an Italy that no longer exists. I think to myself that despite her complaints of the noise and crowds in Rome, at least we won't be in the streets of Napoli anymore. Dad and I had intentionally planned our trip to begin in Milano, figuring we would then work our way down the country, and be more seasoned by the time we arrived in Rome. In fact, if nothing else, by now I notice we have both become bolder at crossing highly-trafficked streets and dodging cars and bicycles. Yesterday, we wandered right out into a wide, crazy, Napolese avenue with our hands in a halt sign. This behavior may be considered gauche in Torino or Milano, but in Napoli where autos and motorcycles fly like bats out of hell it's the only way to cross the sea of never-ending vehicles.

We disembark the Circumvesuviana and wander a distance before we locate Pompeii. I buy a guide book and Dad leaves it up to me to decide what we want to visit. We know nothing about the layout of the destroyed city and attempting to find the best sites within the 160 acres proves challenging. We have no idea what we are looking at as we trudge over thickly cobbled, uneven pathways, through destroyed ruins and gobs of *turisti*. A great surprise, however, is the location of the old city itself, set in a fertile valley surrounded by vineyards and mountains and Vesuvius looming immediately nearby. At one point we wander away from the ruins and relish being the only two people strolling within this serene valley that edges up to the outskirts of Pompeii. Crossing through a park-like setting shaded by a row of towering cypress trees, we emerge onto acres of ripe, plum tomato vines and help ourselves to a great, sugary mid-day snack. We meander back to the ruins, where I resume looking perplexed at the map since we have yet to see any of the great stuff pictured in the guide book: where are the remains of ancient temples and the statues and mosaics still intact? A British woman, who seems to be noticing my growing frustration, interjects facetiously: *"What? You can't figure out an Italian made map?"* Everyone in earshot gets a good laugh out of this, as she sidles up to me and peers over my shoulder at the guide book. *"What exactly do you want to see?"* she asks, helpfully. *"Anything!"* I reply, exasperated. She points me in the direction of the House of Vitti (whatever that is) after which we eventually stumble upon bakeries, community baths, an amphitheatre, temples, homes with fountains and faded frescoes and a number of public laundry spots. We spend time standing within the ruins of a *take-away* food bar where refreshments were once stored in big clay wells built into long tiled counters that remain in tact. The wells of the bar kept food and drinks cool for patrons, such as those who might have just paid a visit to one of the town brothels.

By late afternoon, Dad looks wiped out. We have logged in approximately six, hard miles of trudging along the uneven cobbled pathways of Pompeii. Beginning with our circuitous route this morning to the port of Naples, sitting out a thunder storm, meandering about Sorrento, and more than a miles' jog to the Circumvesuviana train station, we are both beat. In need of a beer and a meal, we head toward the modern town of Pompeii Stavi, which looks an arm's distance away, then turns out to be another mile or more. We pass a bunch of tour buses and pick the first *non-turisti* restaurant we can locate. Immediately, we order two pints of beer, which we quaff with elation. The bread that comes to our table is *panini di pizza* and it's excellent. The general texture resembles that of the pizza dough of Naples, but it is doubled over like a round bun and baked quickly. Ravenous, we begin eating the doughy bread before our meals arrive. The dressing for our salads is olive oil and—instead of the carafe of vinegar—this time we receive a quarter wedge of ripe lime: it's quite good this way. Fresh calamari and the pasta dish we order satisfy our famished bodies.

Back aboard the rickety Circumvesuviana, we continue along the bay and past the destroyed town of Herculeneum, as we continue back to Napoli. The train makes frequent stops so it's easy for cons, beggars and commuters to scam the system, particularly since we notice no conductors passing through to validate tickets. Shortly into our trip, a young Italian woman, cradling a large accordion, jumps on board. With vacuous eyes, she waltzes up to us and taps a few keys, barely squeezing the bellows, producing some lame excuse for a tune. Obviously the accordion is simply a prop for her begging. I don't think she actually knows how to play the instrument. She gives up on us pretty quickly, careens down the isle to a few more commuters and slips off at the next stop.

When we are dumped off at the Napoli station, it's as scary as ever. I slip my neck purse under my shirt and keep a watchful eye on Dad's pack full of rain jackets, umbrellas and my digital camera. One step out of the depot and we're back into the trash laden streets that have become our home base these past three days. The blocks surrounding the station are burgeoning with locals hanging about. We try a new route home, in an attempt to avoid the busy Umberto Corso I. It's impossible not to get disoriented amidst the sea of moving locals. To add to our confusion, the streets fan out in all directions, like the tentacles of a squid, and cars are parked on the sidewalks, as well as double parked in the streets. Dad seems especially nervous as he moves at record speed, stopping every few minutes to look at the map, then moving on again. I'm lagging behind him and he is beginning to take on the appearance of some kind of deranged mosquito, his light frame flitting off the crowds like a tiny pinball. Amidst the mayhem, some Italian guy stops his car, leans out the window and whistles at me, grinning lasciviously. Somehow I am flattered by his crass attention. Maybe I've dropped a few pounds, running around this city, lost, perspiring and frightened to death. With the help of a kindly local, we maneuver our way back towards our hotel. Wading through the littered alleyway, we pass locals buying beer for street parties and kids engaged in a pick-up game of soccer. Families emerge from shops with groceries, and noise resounds from all directions. Naples is wild and crazy, but come to think of it we have witnessed no violence during our stay. Granted, we are careful and take precautions, such as being locked in our room by 7:30 PM, but nonetheless, we have not been accosted or conned or violated in any way.

Safely back in our impregnable fortress, hot showers feel *fantastico*. I turn on the Italian news and see that it's been raining intermittently in Rome the past few days. The broadcast runs a segment on downtown Milano's street side photography exhibit we walked through only days ago. There are clips of the presidential debates back home. The whole world is watching. During our last dinner in Florence, a waiter asked us about Bush. We stuck with our party line: Bush *e molto male!* Our waiter concurred and shook his head muttering something about the war in Iraq.

After a full day of circling the entire south side of the Bay of Napoli, this is the most beat we have been. For the first time on this trip, Dad tells me his feet have grown weary. I manage to suspend from all physical pain, uplifted by the knowledge that this will be our last night in Napoli—the night I have been dreaming of for three days. Tomorrow we will awake and get our sore asses out of this city and head for Rome—the final leg of our Italian journey.

Sore feet are nothing new to me. Day Three—the Trek Team's final ascent to Base Camp—was really challenging. By this time, we had a culmination of three long days of climbing into ever thinning air, through boulder-laden terrain, with 60 mile an hour afternoon winds that blew dirt into our hair, the fibers of our clothing and the creases of our skin. Rest stops came none too soon on the mountain. Just about when I thought I couldn't take another step, Tuck would finally yell out" Rest Break!" and we got relief for a good 20 minutes before we took off again. I remember well our final rest stop, prior to entering Base Camp at 14,000 feet. I released my pack and dropped to the ground next to Dr. Grant. We rested there in silence for awhile, both of us appreciating the spectacular panorama of the Andes before us. She broke the silence when she looked over to me and exclaimed "We did it!" throwing her arms around me in a hearty embrace. "I'll never forget the day I met you in the hospital" she commented. Her statement took me by surprise. Wasn't it I who should remember her? For, I too couldn't forget the day we had met: two of 14 lymph nodes sampled from my armpit proved positive, meaning I would require six months of an aggressive cocktail of chemotherapy, and it was Dr. Grant I had chosen as my oncologist to oversee the treatments. Now that I think about it, I doubt I would have been on this mountain climb had it not been for the serendipity that led me to Dr. Grant. I doubt I would have even heard about Expedition Inspiration or considered tackling such a beast, had it not been for Dr. Grant's encouragement. It moved me now to learn that I had made an impression on her. Perhaps she remembers all her patients, I thought as I considered that she too had struggled with health issues—an unusual cancer of the tongue that usually strikes only smokers and older men. Other emotions surfaced for me that afternoon as we ascended higher in the Andes Range, miles from civilization. Visions of my family and friends appeared—those who had endured the emotional and physical roller coaster ride beside me. I'll never forget the anguished look on my mother's face as she heard the word "aggressive" in reference to my tumor or the heavy weight that was lifted from my entire family when I completed my final round of the toxic chemo—the "cure."

As the Trek Team drew closer to Base Camp that afternoon, I felt extremely proud of our team. After three days of climbing uphill, downhill, gaining and losing in elevation, forging streams, straddling mules, moving against heavy winds and pitching and breaking down tents, at last, we were about to arrive. I felt we had each pulled our individual weight while also cooperating as a team. Not all of the women of Expedition Inspiration were super athletes, many of us were not. Now, despite our previous years of struggling with a life-threatening disease, we seemed to be bouncing back, in a most empowering and positive way. Like stealthy warriors, we walked single file into Base Camp that afternoon, taking our final steps of the three day journey upward. At 14,000 feet we entered a barren moonscape-an expansive mountain basin cradled beneath the shadows of Aconcagua's snowy peak. We were cheered into camp by Jeannie Morris, our documentary producer, who had ascended to Base with the Summit Team several days earlier. A group of other climbers whooped and hollered us into the high mountain basin—our home for the next four nights. Congratulations abounded, as the women of the Trek Team embraced and our film crew of two, kept their cameras rolling. Jeannie passed around a few encouraging notes scribbled by various members of our Summit Team who were now camped at 19,000 feet. That evening at dinner I read one aloud that I had received from Summit member, Claudia Berryman-Shaefer: "I think of all of you all the time ... you're pushing me up the mountain. Kick back and relax, it's awesome here. Celebrate your wellness."

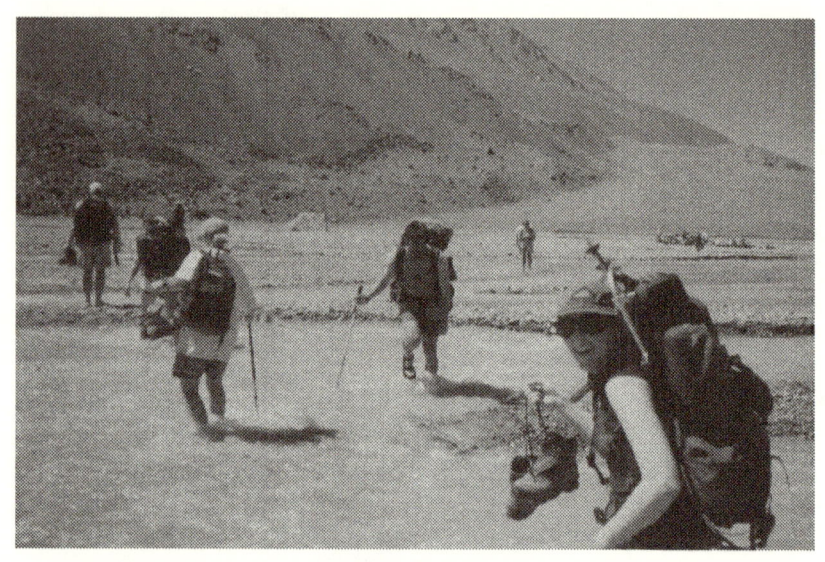

Cold Crossing

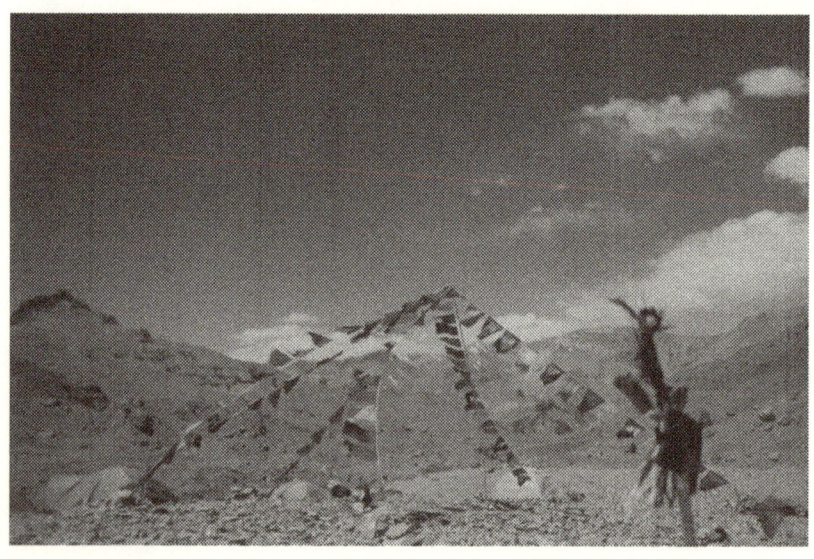

Base Camp

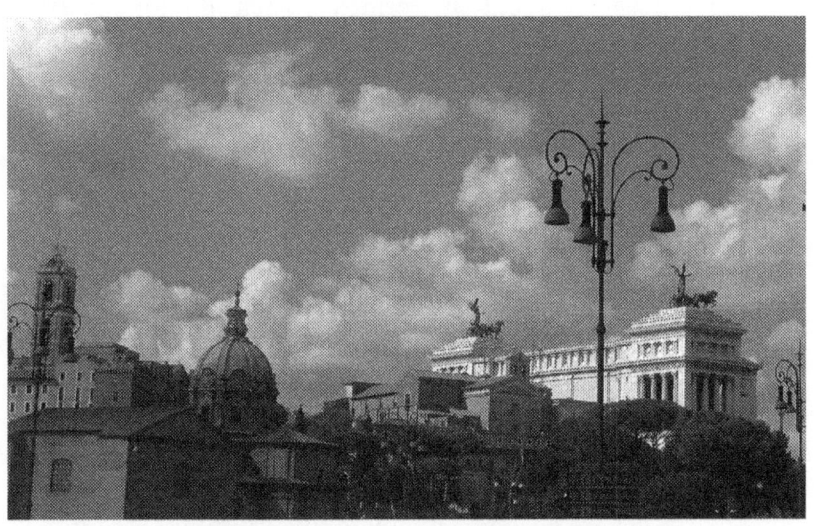

Roma—Backside of the Wedding Cake

Roma

12 Ottobre

It is not the earthy scent of Vernazza's sea air nor the fresh aroma of Milano's baking brioche to which we awake this morning. After early rains, it is the effluence of sewage that greets our olfactory senses. This open-air refuse heap—following a healthy Napoli downpour—has churned up a toxic concoction of urine, dog shit, discarded corn cobs, spilt beer, coke and cigarette butts, to beat the band. *We're outta here!* I put the final punctuation mark in my journal entry, as I sit patiently at attention on the bed waiting for dad to lock his backpack. On our way to the train station, we kick our way through trash and follow groups of youngsters huddled beneath umbrellas presumably on their way to school. Monday morning in Napoli seems calm in comparison to the street chaos of this past weekend. The streets are easier to navigate this morning—the blocks leading to the train station void of barking venders. We stop for our daily cappucino, this time armed with lots of small change drawers. Poor ole' Napoli: all these people seemed to want from us was small enough bills in an effort to avoid wiping out their change. In fact, this was the one thing the locals were adamant about: like some unwritten law in Naples *"smaller change!"* was the mantra of every shop and even at the museum and ferry terminal. Yesterday, while Dad thumbed through a wad of euros that could probably feed a Neopolitan family for three months, I stood by feeling incredibly embarrassed and guilty as accused for being a privileged white American gringa. Regardless of the poor economic conditions of the south, however, from all I have observed in these few days, the Neopolitans go about their lives with no less joy than the other communities we have walked through during our travels. In fact, Napoli is one hell of a spirited city.

Boarding a 9:00 AM train to Rome this morning, we take advantage of the many vacant seats and each settle into our own coach. It isn't long out of Napoli before we reach beautiful countryside— this particular rail following a Mediterranean route. Most of the country we have covered in the past few weeks appears to be well-cultivated in orchards, crops, and vineyards. It seems that almost every strip of land available in Italy is put to good use. Earlier in our travels—near the train tracks of Florence—I was impressed by a well-cared for community garden wedged within a group of humble shacks. On the island of Procida, I observed vegetables growing curbside on slender strips of soil between homes. In Vernazza, homes dotting the mountainsides boasted terraced garden plots of robust vegetables, their vines staked with the local bamboo.

Just north of Naples our train stops and a middle-aged Italian woman boards seating herself in Dad's compartment. In hesitant, broken English, she politely asks Dad if he minds her eating a sandwich. "No" he manages to reply, his tongue incredibly loosened after only two-1/2 weeks in Italy. I overhear her telling him she has been taking English lessons and I can detect she wants to practice her skills on him. Dad is saying: *"mia figlia, mia figlia"* and pointing at me, as I write in my journal. I lift my head and nod in confirmation: "Si!", "I am his daughter." She is telling him that she is a professor and is on her way to Formia, perhaps to a workshop. We also learn that she has a daughter living in Spain. Dad's doing his best to communicate, and I notice both of them glancing over to me for help. I decide to join in the conversation and explain that my great-grandparents were from the Piedmont region and had immigrated to the US in the early 1900's. She shakes her head, lamenting the many Italians who had emigrated from the country following the war. When our train reaches Formia, I note its pleasant seaside location and think it might be a nice off-the-beaten location, should I ever travel this way again. The woman seems quite pleased to have had a successful exchange with *l'Americani*. We smile *"Arrivederci"* wishing we knew how to say more and she in turn departs with some Italian salutation that we think might have meant *have a good day* or *Have a good time in Roma*.

By the time our train arrives into the station at Rome, we are elated to emerge onto spotlessly clean, wide city sidewalks. A crisp, cool late morning air greets us and high, dramatic clouds float within rain-cleansed skies. We are barely away from the train station when already we know we are going to love this city. We share the sidewalks with an unbelievably sparse number of pedestrians. Our gait feels lighter, and smiles brighten our travel-weary faces as we jaunt toward our last *albergo*. We are no longer in the litter-strewn streets of Napoli or the closed-in mazes of Firenze or Venizia. Rome feels open, expansive, visually stimulating and above all else … it's CLEAN! Missing Rome's summer tourist season and hot spells undoubtedly will make our stay more pleasant. For us, Rome is like a breath of fresh air—like the icing on the cake.

Our hotel, The Monti Residence, is located in a great neighborhood on a short street, called Via Serpenti, and located within easy walking distance of the Coliseum. Across the street from our new digs is an inviting coffee bar managed by a gregarious woman who bustles about keeping her patrons happy. A barista juggles numerous customers with experience and ease. Next door to the coffee bar is a *gelateria* offering 75 flavors. Down the street is a lavenderia, which we need to use for the last time in our travels: this one is drop-off and pick up the next day for 10 Euro—a nice break from self-service. The restaurants on Via Serpenti are predominantly East Indian. We notice small shops selling East Indian nick nacks and clothing. A produce stand, a farmacia, a hair salon and the like, are among the businesses that line this short city block. In the days to come, I notice locals milling about—many of them stopping to chat—a common past-time of *l'italiani*. I remember how curious I was when in our Italian language class spent time learning how to conjugate the verb "to chat." I am curious no more, as after almost three weeks in Italy I understand how truly integral chatting is to this culture—chatting, hanging out, gesticulating, embracing, singing, promenading, shouting, screaming—the world is vibrantly alive and well in the streets of Italy.

After settling into our room, we head straight for the Coliseum. Circling the outside of the ruins, we decide to visit the interior early some other day when we are feeling fresh and the crowds are thinner. We mosey through the Forum and past the Arch of Constantine—the stretch of Imperial Roman ruins that Rick Steve's refers to as *Caesar's Shuffle*. At our feet lie big chunks of toppled white marble Corinthian columns, patterned in fleur-de-lis and others with Roman letters and numerals. The magnificent rubble is preserved as a national monument that rests in the heart of the city amidst modern, medieval and renaissance Rome. We ramble onward into another architectural era altogether as we reach the backside of a monolithic, solid white marble monument that seems to occupy about a city block. My eyes are riveted upward to the rooftop where two winged goddesses driven by chariots blend into a spectacular backdrop of floating clouds. It occurs to me we are staring at the backside of what is commonly referred to in Italy as the *wedding cake*—a massive monument built to commemorate Italy's unification of 1865. It is dedicated to Vittorio Emmanuelle II, the first king of the united country. Other nicknames adopted to describe its architecture are *la macchina da scrivere* (the typewriter) and *the dentures*. The monument serves no function other than symbolic and takes up a great deal of space overwhelming everything in proximity. Although over the years, this architecture has met with some harsh criticism, Dad and I rather like it and in the days to come it serves as a great landmark to keep us oriented.

Rome is a great walking city. In two hours we have wandered through Imperial Roman ruins, a medieval village and architecture of more modern times. I see now why it is referred to as a city of many layers. We roam through neighborhoods of piazzas, past churches and shops, until we begin to notice crowds gathered in the area of the Trevi Fountain and Spanish Steps. Unlike Florence—where it seemed impossible to escape the tourist-packed streets—we are finding in Rome we can easily duck away from a tourist attraction into a less-crowded area. After a late lunch in a cafeteria (the cafeterias of Rome being really quite good) we commence with our usual wandering about and don't arrive back to Via Serpenti until late in the day. I fantasize about returning to Rome some year and planting myself here for a good solid month, giving me enough time to explore more thoroughly and at a relaxed pace.

My travels of recent years have been anything but relaxed. The day following the Trek Team's arrival to Base Camp had been set aside as a "rest day." Some rest! Nancy and I commiserated as we gathered boulders and constructed a two foot high rock wall around our tent to fortify it against fierce evening winds. The film crew insisted on group shots of us sporting our gear from numerous sponsors, that afternoon. For the first time on the mountain, I felt drained and lethargic from the high altitude. I was unmotivated to do a thing. Some of my team mates, however, were more spirited: they spent some time erecting a maypole of prayer flags in the center of our tent sites. Colorful streams of orange, magenta, teal blue and red flags festooned downward like a circus tent from a central post and anchored to the rocks below. In the late afternoon, I could hear the cotton flags flapping madly in the wind. Inscribed upon each bright square were the words: "May the winds bring healing. May the winds bring serenity and remembrance. May we be free from illness." The following morning we formed a circle and held hands around the maypole. Each woman, mountain guide, doctor and member of our team, acknowledged a special person and paid tribute to each other. We considered our Summit Team members holed up in their tents at 19,000 feet waiting out another snow storm. The next good weather day they would attempt the summit, waking around 3:00 AM, roped together in teams of four and five, and prepared to make the assault by 5:00 AM. In one long, brutal day they would climb from 19,000 to the 23,000 feet, returning back to High Camp before dusk. Two Summit members had already turned back and descended to Base Camp: both Andrea Gabbard, our team writer, and Mary Yeo, from Portland, Maine, had "hit the wall" at 19,000 feet. The wise thing to do when you feel really ill on the mountain is to descend. Although Andrea and Mary appeared to be physi-

cally spent and understandably disappointed, they were happy to be greeted by the smiling faces of the Trek Team back at Base. They took advantage of foot massages, provided by Sue Anne, our self-appointed masseuse. On rest day, Sue Anne had painted a pair of wandering feet and the words" Massage Parlor— Bring Your Feet Here" on the outside of her tent. Sue Anne had become infamous in the past year for hauling loads of her "stuff" on our practice climbs. On Aconcagua she lugged along a video camera, a set of paints, massage lotion, tarot cards and a kite that she flew in the late afternoon winds at Base Camp. I can still picture her out on a precipice, the rainbow colored kite spiraling upwards within the mountain range. I wonder how Sue Anne would fare with a 12 lb. limit on a trip to Italy. Something tells me she would rise to the occasion.

I can feel Dad and I are slowing down our pace. We have experienced a great deal in the past three weeks, and our feet are beginning to rebel. These last two days we'll take our time and try to savor each final hour in Italy. I long to venture out at least one evening and see if the old rubble and monuments are lit up at night. When Dad gets home with the laundry this evening, we do exactly that and discover that Rome by night is quite lovely.

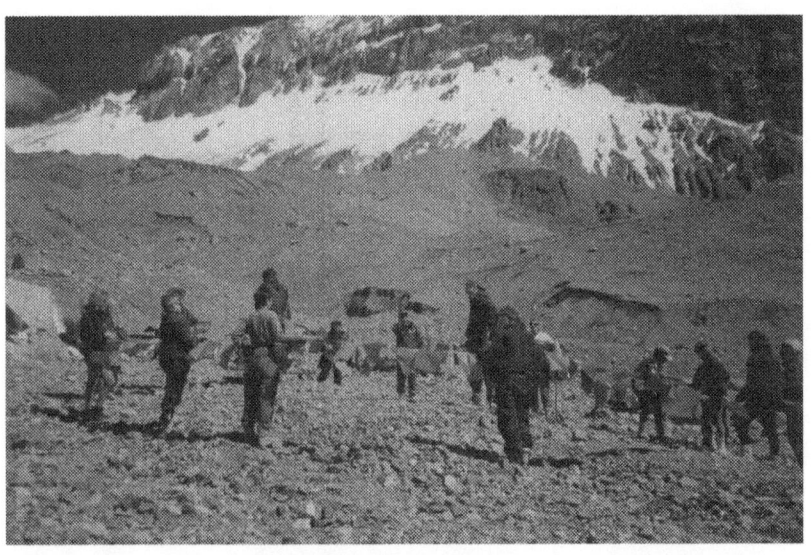

Morning Ceremony

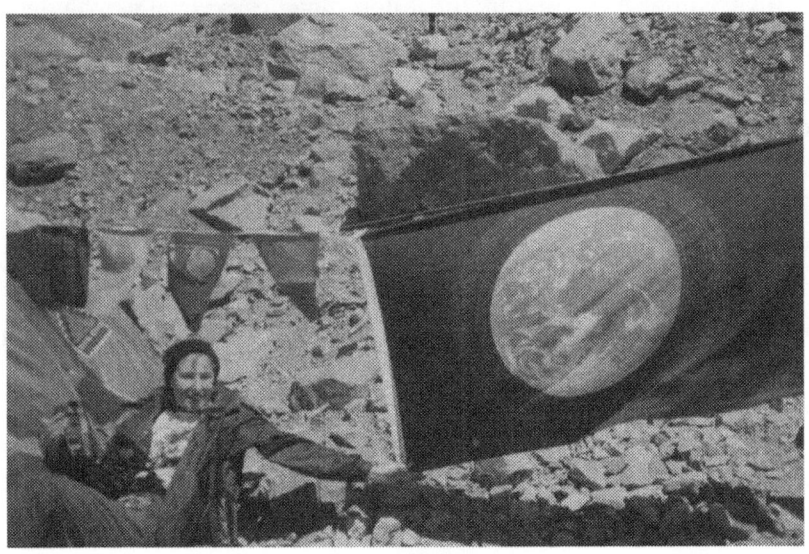

Sue Anne

13 Ottobre

The Sistine Chapel, located beside the Vatican Museum, is one destination we are both in agreement is worth a wait in line to see. We'll need to arrive there by 8:00 AM, so Dad suggests we do a trial-run of Rome's subway today in preparation for the real deal tomorrow morning. We study the map and determine a walking route through unexplored neighborhoods for our trek back home from Vatican City. Our loop today will include a stroll by the Piazza Navona and The Pantheon. With cappucino stops, a long, leisurely lunch and our requisite gelato break, we figure this will make a full day.

Rome's Metro has only two lines because further subterranean expansion would mean unearthing and disturbing a city full of ruins. As a result, the lines that do exist are crowded. Studying the map of the Metro stations, Dad zeroes in on the closest stop to our hotel, determines on which side of the rail we must be positioned, at which stop to transfer and where to disembark in order to be in the closest proximity to the Vatican Museum. Finding the metro stop this morning, however, takes some trial and error, so our practice run is already proving to be a wise decision. Once inside Rome's subway station, we have difficulty determining what tickets to purchase and from which of the many machines. A young Italian man—noticing our confusion—comes to our rescue. Communicating through pantomime, he helps us buy tickets and leads us through turnstiles where we join a stream of commuters. Like a school of lemmings, en masse we serpentine quickly down flights of stairs and round corners until we disappear into the claustrophobic tunnel below. Our young guide to the underground leaves us at the platform. In my hurry I don't realize that perhaps he was expecting a tip. Instead, he receives grateful smiles as Dad and I nervously wedge within dozens of commuters.

When the train arrives we can see it is packed shoulder to shoulder with people. Dad must have some experience with crowded subways, for the moment the doors of the car open, rather than wait for another perhaps less-crowded car to arrive, he aggressively shoves me into the hordes as the door slams shut behind us. We stand erect like canned sardines, as I grab an overhead rail with one hand and protect my neck purse with the other. In all our travels throughout Italy, this is the most uncomfortable and claustrophobic I have felt. My face feels flush from a sudden hot flash and I think I might faint, something I have never before experienced. Why not simply take a cab to the Vatican tomorrow—I ask myself— then I realize this would ruin Dad's fun. I think he gets a thrill from overcoming transportation hurdles. Once we successfully arrive near Vatican City, we walk another 20 minutes before we find the Vatican Museum. By 10:30 this morning I notice there is already a line of about 50 people at the entrance. We agree that a 6:30 AM wakeup call tomorrow is a must.

We enjoy wandering the open streets of Rome today. Bernini's exquisite, marbled fountains in the Piazza Navona are the work of a true master and the interior of The Pantheon, with its multi-hued and patterned marble design, is another impressive architectural feat. A young American student and instructor of English as a Second Language, who is on leave from her work in Seoul, tags along with us for awhile. We buy a gelato together and talk about the ease of getting around Rome. Perhaps it is due to the fact that we are traveling on the "shoulder" of the tourist season that our waltz through Rome seems so crowd-free. With a few intermittent showers, a late lunch break in a warm osteria is welcomed. I savor a slow roasted lamb shank with rosemary, a regional specialty. It's excellent alongside a heap of piping hot spinach. After lunch, we stroll by a medieval castle and village that flank several city blocks. Constructed from thin red bricks, some of the medieval buildings actually used the existing columns of Imperial Roman ruins as partial support—a visual testimony to the many layers of the city. Below our feet lies a world we will not even see. I read in a National Geographic article I found at our hotel in Florence, that below Imperial Rome lays Phoenician Rome, but in order not to disturb the Roman ruins Phoenicia remains beneath the city, untouched. We pause to admire a colony of well-fed feral cats that live within a fenced-in section of Imperial Roman ruins. The felines disappear and reappear from within their subterranean habitat, which no doubt provides sufficient warmth in the winter, as well as a cool refuge in the heat of the summer. Next to the ruins, a sign in Italian reads something like: *Please do not feed this colony of cats. They are well cared for. If you want to help the gatti please make a donation at such and such an address.* I am impressed, once again, and moved by the compassionate people of Rome who have obviously made good use of the ruins as a natural habitat for the feral cats.

With only two days remaining on our trip, I notice my journal entries are becoming a tad gloomy. I am not looking forward to returning to the grind of my job and the stuffy, windowless office environment, especially after three weeks of outdoor walking in Italy. It amazes me the engineers who do not consider natural light and fresh air when designing buildings. I am finding it difficult at mid-life to consider leaving my retirement plan early, yet the thought of facing ten more years of the same repetitive work is taking it's toll on my mind, body and spirit. I have always found my outlets for creativity, intellectual stimulation and personal growth, outside of my job. Now, as I gear up for my return home, these issues begin to weigh on me again. Suspending from this anxiety about my work life these past three weeks has been as therapeutic as stepping outside of the American culture altogether. I love waking each morning to a new adventure. I felt that way about Expedition Inspiration. Knowing I would spend nine days in the great outdoors with fresh air and a community of friends was far better therapy than I could possibly receive from a prescription drug or a counseling sessions. Knowing for two weeks my eyes would rest on mountain vistas, my feet would touch the earth and my mind could unwind during long stretches of silence was just what the doctor ordered.

February 4, 1995 was Summit Day for Expedition Inspiration. The previous night, Tuck had asked the Trek Team for a show of hands from those desiring to challenge themselves to ascend to 19,000 feet. Many of us were in greater physical condition than ever before in our lives and it was tempting to see what existed higher up the mountain. Andrea Gabbard had encouraged Nancy and me to climb to 19,000 feet, simply to feel the beauty of the snow-covered Andes Range from that perspective. I think from peer pressure I must have raised my hand, because in all honesty I was daunted by an uphill gain of 5,000 feet in one day, especially as it fell on the highly-anticipated day of the summit assault. I was, therefore, not altogether disappointed when our sojourn was abruptly aborted the following morning. At 5:30 AM as Nancy and I emerged from our tent, clothed in layer upon layer of gear, Tuck accosts us with the news that our team nurse, Saskia, had pulmonary edema. "Nobody's going up to 19,000 feet today," he announced, "I'm sending Ned back down the mountain with Saskia. This is going to put us out one mountain guide and we can't afford for anything more to happen, especially on Summit Day. If a group of you wants to take a shorter climb today, instead, I have no problem with that." Ironically, Saskia is a nurse, and one who seems to take care of herself last. She had come into the expedition with a head cold, which had grown into a whooping cough by the time we reached 14,000 feet. With our mission to 19,000 feet abandoned, our intrepid group lingered over a leisurely breakfast of bagels and coffee, and decided to take a trek to 15,500 feet that day instead. The ascent was harder than I expected. The breathing was harder, the climbing much steeper than before and we were now entering heavy snow pack. The vistas were growing grander, as well, and for that it was worth it. As we continued upward, the view of our campsite in the basin below grew smaller. From a precipice, we could barely make out the maypole of prayer flags and orange Jansport tents that were now swallowed within the vast range of the Andes. By mid-day, we passed the penitentes, an expansive and other-worldly looking snow field of ice pinnacles that seemed frozen in suspended animation. At noon we reached a serene, snowy mountain basin where we lounged against boulders for over an hour in the sun, resting and eating canned sardines, crackers and cheese. It must have been about 1:00 pm when two of our summit team members, Annette Porter and Paul DeLorey, descended from the trail above us on their way back down to Base Camp. They both looked spaced out and could barely muster up words as it became clear to us they had to turn back at some point from the summit attempt. Their faces expressed disappointment and we didn't press them for details. Our group arrived back at Base Camp that afternoon around 4:00 PM. We spotted the rest of the team huddled together on a plateau facing the summit of Aconcagua. Our mountain guide, Erika Whitakker, held a short-wave radio, waiting to hear from husband, Peter, who had been leading the summit team on the ascent that day. We raced over to join the rest of the team as the afternoon winds by now had picked up force. By 4:30 we got the call: "Base, this is the summit team. Do you copy?" Peter's voice crackled across the air waves. "The Trek Team is all here!" Erika screamed back, excitedly. "We're facing the peak of the mountain!" We could hear Peter's voice yelling back that the team was about 150 feet from reaching the summit. "We're gonna make it!" he screamed, as team members on all sides of me broke out in yelps and tears of joy. Then, in syncopated unison, we began blowing forceful pressure breaths into the microphone of the radio as if spiriting the summit team up the final leg of their journey. Minutes later we could make out shrieks— the voices of Laura Evans, Claudia Berryman-Shaefer, Nancy Knoble, Dr. Bud Alpert and Peter Whitakker: "We made it!" one of them shouted, the sounds of their voices all but obscured by the afternoon winds. "It's unbelievable up here!"

We learned later that the last six hours of the ascent were brutal. It didn't help matters that their morning had begun with the first rope team falling shoulder and waist deep into a snowy pit. This gobbled up a great deal of energy and time required to flail themselves back out. Some of the team, such as Annette, never quite recovered and eventually had to turn back in order for the others to press ahead. The Summit Team traversed the glacier for several more hours in the pitch dark that morning, freezing and uncomfortable, until day break. The most difficult terrain of the assault lay hours ahead of them with the final ascent of the dreaded "Cantaletta"—the rock-laden peak. One step upward and ten steps back on the talus, scree and snow seemed to be the climbing norm on this final leg of the slag heap. By this point, climbing was slow going and rest stops were required every twenty minutes to catch their breath. Most of them didn't remember much from those final hours as their senses had become obscured within a blinding world of whiteness and their minds by now had turned to mush. Three of the women of Expedition Inspiration reached the 23,000 ft peak that afternoon, yet it was the concerted energy and teamwork of all that made this a lasting and enriching journey. We all spirited the team up that afternoon. With the summit assault behind us, we could now let down our guard and relax. The next day-Feb. 5th-the entire team would reunite physically for the first time on mountain. February 5th also marked my 42nd birthday. I had much to celebrate.

14 Ottobre

After a 6:30 A.M. wake up call, by 9:00 o'clock we are quietly seated on a bench inside the Sistine Chapel taking in Michelangelo's beautiful painted ceiling of rich gold, blues and sepia. In silence, I study the sensual soft faces and perfectly foreshortened figures painted within the arched corners. The chapel is not too lousy with *turisti* yet. We had been advised by a friend that as soon as we enter the Vatican Museum to immediately make a beeline to the opposite end where the Chapel is located. Once we visit the chapel we would then work our way backwards through the Museum to the front entrance.

On our return back through the Museum, we are ecstatic not to be a part of one of the numerous tour groups huddled together, listening to a guide wax on about a particular piece of art. The Vatican Museum is immense, so I zero in on the Raphael Rooms to take a look at the *School of Athens,* among other works of the master. After the Raphael Rooms, we move against a swelling tide of tourists, stopping occasionally to admire intricate tapestries, ancient maps and many more marble torsos. The Vatican Museum houses a comprehensive collection of antiquities, and I realize we will need to pare our visit down to no more than two hours, for that is about when Dad's museum buzzer sounds off. Dizziness and fatigue begin to overtake his entire being as he quickly descends into "museum burnout". We spend the remainder of our time on the lower floor marveling at the Egyptian collection of well-preserved mummies and sarcophagi. Painted in brilliant pigments, the interiors of wooden coffins are inscribed with detailed animal motifs, scarabs, and dogs: the personal guides to the underworld. As I predicted, we do the entire museum in a hair less than two hours. I am just as ready as Dad to leave the tourist attraction, in need of fresh air and a cappucino bar. By now, our bodies have grown quite stiff after a three-week culmination of pounding the varied pavements of Italy.

We have lunch today at a cafeteria where we order grilled vegetables and fresh pesto pasta. This is the only incident during our travels that our hostess is aggressively seeking customers off the street. Like a barker, she follows us from outside the restaurant, leads us to a glass-enclosed food counter, and begins translating our meal selections to an overweight Italian woman who serves up hot food from big trays. The female barker begins suggesting additional dishes and requests a quart of beer for each of us, instead of the pint size that we had asked for. *"No!"* I adamantly shake my head, repeating that we both prefer the pint size and that we are contented with the quantity of our meals. *"I feel sorry for her"* Dad tells me later. *"It must be a tough way to make a living."* We top off our daily wanderings this afternoon with delicious gelato from the gelateria across from our hotel.

February 5th was the day following Summit Day for Expedition Inspiration. I was greeted by sunny skies and the sounds of my teammates singing "Happy Birthday" at the cook tent that morning. Using color crayons and her saliva, Kim painted a birthday card for me of our orange Jansport tents nestled in the moonscape of Basecamp, capturing the beautiful palate of the Andes Range. Half of the Trek Team remained at Base Camp that day, preparing for our evening reunion celebration. The rest of us climbed to 16,250 feet to meet up with the Summit team and help carry gear back down. We climbed past the snowfield of ice pinnacles and beyond the big basin in which we took lunch the previous day. The final 500 feet that day were grueling: it felt like straight up snow, ice, scree and talus. Now I was truly getting a taste of what mountain climbing was all about. When we finally reached Camp I, we were greeted by an elated summit team and "Happy Birthday" was sung to me for a second time that day—this time, at 16,250 feet in the Andes, my highest point ever. We helped pack gear down to Base and by the afternoon were at last reunited as a team. That evening our reunion celebration began with a feast of spaghetti and French bread and two altitude-challenged, no-bake cheese cakes prepared lovingly by our mountain guides. Laura, Peter and Tuck cracked open bottles of champagne and surprised us with a boom box and music they had packed up on one of the mules. Earlier that day, while I was making the climb up to 16,250 feet, Kim and Patty were back at Base Camp designing a hideous birthday gown for me—the remnants of a tent that had been left at Base after being blown apart earlier in heavy winds. In honor of my birthday, they tied me up in a toga of tarp, the Expedition

Inspiration logo felt-penned across the bodice and a small bungee cord bracelet accessorizing my wrist. Other "surprises" and stories were shared among the reunited team that evening. The piece-de-resistance, however, came compliments of Annette and Eleanor who emerged from a Jansport tent dressed in slinky cocktail dresses, high heels and chartreuse wigs, gyrating to the raucous bellowing of Tina Turner's "What's Love Got to Do with It?!". Actually, love's got a lot to do with it, I thought, as I looked around at my teammates who by now were dancing and celebrating our successful journey. Beneath a canopy of stars, few souls could hear us as we danced into the night—the women, the men, the mountain guides, the doctors, the photographers, all of us together, exhausted and exhilarated, one big happy family. I knew this was going to be a birthday to beat all birthdays and one that I would not soon forget.

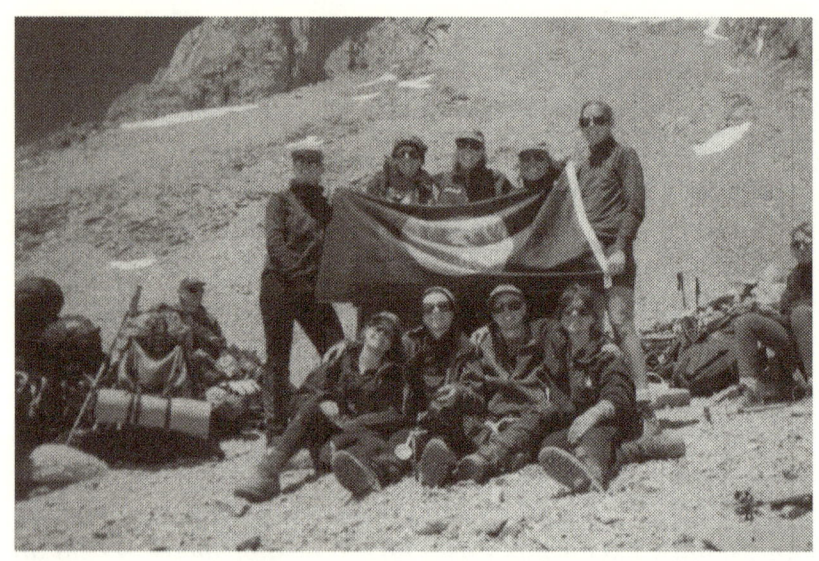

Teams Meet at Camp I—16,250 ft.

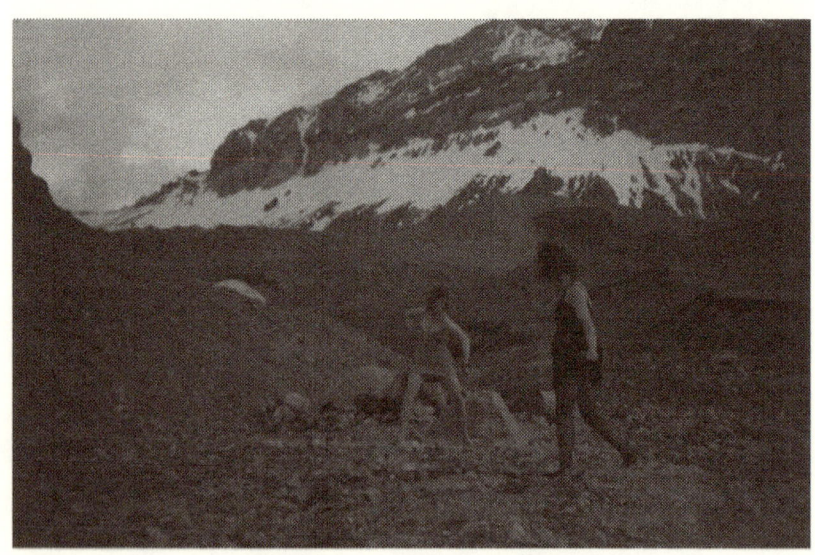

What's Love Got to Do with It?

15 Ottobre

This morning will be our last *capuccini e brioche*. We slowly savor the warm brew at a table in the coffee bar located across from our hotel. For the last time, we enjoy the bustle of locals who pop in and out for a quick espresso before beginning their work day. We leisurely wander over to the Coliseum and notice a scarcity of tourists at this early hour. We spend time exploring the inside of the ruins, and ramble about an upper level where we discover an impressive exhibit—a continuous, long, plasma screen that twists through the marbled columns of the Coliseum, displaying ongoing film footage of the initial unearthing of rubble and the history and preservation of the ruins. The entire floor is darkened to circumvent any glare and marble busts and statues are illuminated by neon blue up-lighting.

We cruise within Cesaer's Shuffle again, taking time to examine the extraordinary pieces of toppled columns decorated with lion's heads, laurel wreathes and fig leaves. I can't seem to get enough of this eye candy. We cross a bridge spanning the Tibre over to the Travestere District, which turns out to be a great, sprawling neighborhood of homes, parks, cathedrals, shops and particularly good looking restaurants. We haven't been successful in the past two nights at finding great Italian food in our neighborhood: the Travestere District, however, looks like the ticket. Numerous *osterias* line one of the streets and sandwich boards boast five and six course meals. We decide to return later, and then amble over to rest our legs for awhile in a church. A rain shower has commenced, so we are not alone as we dart with others into the quiet and warm sanctuary of *Santa Maria in Travestere*. This is the last church we will visit in Italy, so we take our time. The cathedral is unique with its exquisitely-tiled mosaics of gold leaf and bright colors illustrating scenes from the bible. Dad rests in a central wooden pew as I loiter around the periphery of the cathedral admiring the beautiful altars. A brilliant burst of sunlight breaks through the windows, brightening the interior of the cathedral, suddenly. When I return to the pew in which Dad is still seated, he gushes: "Did you get to see the gold-leaf tiles of the walls illuminate when the sun burst through?" "Darn, I missed it" I respond, disappointed, yet happy at Dad's lucky timing having witnessed this visual feast in our final cathedral.

This afternoon in Rome feels beautiful to me. Morning showers are replaced by cool breezes and high dramatic clouds. After a leisurely lunch, we stroll back over one of the arching bridges that cross the Tiber River and make a final, farewell promenade through the layers of ancient, medieval and modern Rome. We relax for a spell in front of the magnificent Arch of Constantine and I stoop to stroke my last Coliseum cat, uncertain if I will ever return. The flying women atop the gargantuan wedding cake rise above us ever-majestic against billowing clouds on this balmy day. Our walks in Rome have been many and varied and I think this one through the Travestere and one last time down the *Caesar Shuffle* are a grand way to end our self-guided tour. We each toss a coin in a fountain and savor our last gelato: this time we both chose a simple ½ crema, ½ cioccolato. *Fantastico!*

There have been times during this trip when I wish I could take a feeling that has overcome me and bottle it, like a drug, for future use. Like the elation I felt as we strolled that first afternoon in Venice along the Giudecca Canale and getting lost within the quiet ancient maze of decay with its hidden gardens and lapping canals. Or the moment the afternoon sun spread a mellow pink wash across a patina green statue in an ancient garden of Pompeii.

Or sitting in the piazetta across from Anna Maria's pensione, enjoying the good air where the sea meets the rich, alluvial soil.

We haven't stayed in three or four or five star hotels, nor have we relaxed within the security of an American tour group, and I think because of this we have gotten a little closer to the Italian people and opened ourselves to some good 'ole serendipity along the way. It is hard to sort out all my feelings and impressions after only three weeks of my initiation to the European culture, but from what I can see, Italy's got a lot of soul. I see it in her architecture and within the charming old downtowns. It exists in the fresh and delicious food. It lies within the vitality of the street life, with its ongoing daily human exchange, where teenagers of the same gender walk arm in arm and people break out into song from time to time. In the streets of Italy I got to know my Dad better and I was visited by a young girl of six and a bright eyed 21 year old who once embraced her world unabashedly as if there was no tomorrow. I believe we all need to suspend and reflect from time to time. My step is feeling a bit lighter now, and who knows—maybe I've unloaded a few rocks from my pockets along the way.

978-0-595-43844-0
0-595-43844-X